Marco Heleno Barreto

PSYCHOLOGY AND THE IRRELE-VANTIFICATION OF MAN

From Jung's project to the post-human times

DUSK OWL BOOKS
London, Ontario, Canada

A publication of

The International Society for Psychology as the Discipline of Interiority

Monograph Series, vol. 4

ISBN 978-1-9992266-4-0

To Teodora

Table of Contents

Sources and Abbreviations

The following abbreviations have been used for frequently cited sources:

CEP: Wolfgang Giegerich. *The Collected English Papers of Wolfgang Giegerich*, 6 vols. New Orleans: Spring Journal Books, 2005-2013. Cited by volume and page number.

WIS: Wolfgang Giegerich. *What is Soul?* New Orleans: Spring Journal Books, 2012. Cited by page number.

CW: Carl Gustav Jung. *Collected Works*, 20 vols. Ed. Herbert Read, Michael Fordham, Gerhard Adler and William McGuire. Trans. R.F.C. Hull. Princeton: Princeton University Press, 1957-1979. Cited by volume and paragraph number.

MDR: Carl Gustav Jung. *Memories, Dreams, Reflections*. Rev. ed., Ed. Aniela Jaffé. Trans. Richard and Clara Winston. New York: Vintage Books, 1989. Cited by page number.

Preface

This book deals with a subject that gradually imposed itself upon me while I was meditating on Wolfgang Giegerich's *The End of Meaning and the Birth of Man*. This subject is the irrelevantification of Man as autonomous and reflective subjectivity in the Age of Technique. The fateful event of emancipation from the soul—from soul as it was known in religion, myth, tradition and classical metaphysics—has not only inaugurated modernity and the correspondent new logical status of modern consciousness, it has paradoxically also rendered human subjectivity psychologically irrelevant (considering the dimension of the logic ruling the objective systems of the world in modernity), so that the birth of Man (as a subject emancipated from soul) is equivalent to the end of Man (as a psychologically relevant agent in soul's *opus magnum*).

This realization led me to examine Jung's psychological project from the perspective of its essential commitment to a specific notion of Man, an ideal of human flourishing embodied in the conception of the process of individuation. I tried to establish, within the lived psychological experience out of which Jung devised his Analytical Psychology, the limits and horizon within which it was proposed. This is the origin of the reflection presented in the first chapter; "Requiem for Analytical Psychology. A reflection on Jung's (Anti)Catastrophic Psychology".[1] The

[1] Originally published in the *Journal of Analytical Psychology*, 2014, 59, 60-77. The version presented here has been revised and modified.

catastrophic aspect or event alluded to in this title, and examined and interpreted in Jung's catastrophic visions and dreams, is precisely the catastrophe of the notion of Man resultant from his emancipation from soul, the catastrophe nested in modernity: the fatal blow on the humanist ideals that constituted the horizon within which Jung's psychology was born and to whose predicament it was addressed.

Jung's idea of individuation was explicitly raised against the simultaneously historical and logical situation assigned to born man in the wider sphere of soul's *opus magnum* after the event of emancipation from soul, namely, the situation of *Vermassung* (massification). Mass Man is thus the surrogate of the autonomous reflective subject in the new order established and gradually unfolded and implemented after the Industrial Revolution. This led me to examine more attentively the definitional features and the process of production of Mass Man and mass-mindedness. In chapter two I present a brief phenomenological description of Mass Man, and then I track its logical roots, from a historical-philosophical perspective, in order to understand the riddle of modernity. This riddle may be expressed this way: modernity produces a one of a kind form of subjectivity and at the same time produces its obliteration. I hope that this attempt at presenting and clarifying this riddle may help to understand what is at stake in Jung's project as well as in our present situation.

To illustrate this situation, which could be called post-Jungian (in the sense implied in the "*Requiem* for Analytical Psychology"), in chapter three I proceed to a detailed interpretation of a contemporary dream, considering it from the perspective of psychology as the discipline of interiority. My intention is to show how the post-human mode of consciousness (correlative of the final triumph of Mass Man in medial modernity) can acquire meaning and purpose, when envisaged as an inescapable moment of a truly modern consciousness engaged with the challenging task of creating a human form of living within a post-human world.[2]

The reader will certainly note the deep and enthusiastic indebtedness of my reflections to Wolfgang Giegerich's psychological thought. I would like to express my gratitude to him for his always kind, forthright and generous support to my theoretical experiments with psychology as the discipline of interiority, while I was in the process of absorbing its principles and methodological approach. I would also like to thank my friend and colleague Greg Mogenson for the inestimable support in the production of this book.

Belo Horizonte, Autumn 2020

---

[2] Part of Chapter 3 ("The End of Man Manifested in Soul's *opus parvum*") has been presented at the Second International Conference of the ISPDI (International Society for Psychology as the Discipline of Interiority), held in Berlin, from 19 to 21 of July, 2014. I would like to express my gratitude to FAPEMIG (Fundação de Amparo à Pesquisa do Estado de Minas Gerais) and to CAPES (Coordenação de Aperfeiçoamento de Pessoal de Nível Superior) for the concession of financial support which allowed me to attend to the Berlin Conference.

Chapter 1

Requiem for Analytical Psychology

A reflection on Jung's (anti)catastrophic psychology

Prolegomenon: Methodological, Conceptual and Theoretical Framework

Küsnacht, 1961: on the eve of his death, Jung has a catastrophic vision depicting the last fifty years of humanity. One of his daughters took notes of the contents of the vision, and afterwards gave them to Marie-Louise von Franz, who kept them in a drawer.[3]

Forty eight years earlier, on October 1913, while on a train journey, Jung had had a twice repeated vision, in which a monstrous flood covered all the northern and low-lying lands between the North Sea and the Alps—mighty yellow waves with the rubble of civilization and the drowned bodies of uncounted thousands—, only countered by the rising mountains which protected Switzerland from the catastrophe, and then the whole sea turned into blood.[4] In the first half of 1914, Jung had three dreams of similar catastrophic contents, with the difference that now an increasing Arctic cold wave covered Europe, devastating all life.

---

[3] See von Franz' interview at the end of the documentary *Matter of Heart*, directed by Mark Whitney, conceived and written by Suzanne Wagner, first released on 22 October 1986.

[4] Jung, *MDR*, p. 175.

In what follows I will examine Jung's catastrophic visions and dreams adopting a very specific interpretative position, anchored in the viewpoint of psychology as the discipline of interiority, which considers a psychic phenomenon *as* meaning itself, being its own interpretation, so that interpreting it is an "attempt to discover the interpretation as which the [psychic phenomenon] *is*".[5] This statement is identical with Jung's position concerning the dream being its own interpretation (see *CW* 11 § 41).[6]

What Jung says about the dream can be extended to all psychological phenomena, which are then taken purely as expressions or statements of "the soul's speaking to itself about itself",[7] and thus as not pointing to anything else but themselves. This does not mean that soul has absolutely no relation to reality. The point here is *methodological*: "Soul-making cannot focus on the individual and it cannot focus on the world. It has to focus on the soul itself, that is, on the logic that is neither, but is the innermost life of both".[8] The *interiorization* of a given phenomenon in itself, leading to the disclosure of its logical life, is thus the aim of the methodological standpoint foundational for psychology as the discipline of interiority.

It should be emphasized that this methodology is grounded in Jung himself. Its basis is the interpretative principle of any psychological phenomenon, established by Jung in these terms: "Above all, don't let anything from outside, that does not belong, get into it, for the fantasy-

---

[5] Giegerich, *CEP III*, p. 180.
[6] See also *C.G. Jung Letters*. Vol. 2. Ed. Gerhard Adler. Princeton: Princeton University Press, 1976, p. 294.
[7] Giegerich, *CEP III*, p. 176.
[8] Giegerich, *CEP III*, p. 249.

image has 'everything it needs' " (*CW* 14 § 749). Giegerich only radicalizes this stance, excluding other principles also admitted by Jung, and thus he creates the methodological profile of a particular psychological approach. This profile is not a personal possession of Giegerich, but an objective and legitimate way of proceeding psychologically. This is the methodological stance adopted in the following reflection.

In using the word "soul", I follow first of all Jung, who abundantly uses *Seele* in his writings. The English translator of the *Collected Works* has opted for the less "scandalous" *psyche*, and this option may have many consequences for the understanding of the deeper nature of Jung's thought, inasmuch as it tends to reduce his psychological project to a problematic *scientific* status,[9] whereas Jung himself saw clearly that psychology "is doomed to cancel itself out as a science [*muß sich als Wissenschaft selber aufheben*] and therein precisely it reaches its scientific goal" (*CW* 8 § 429). One can say that for Jung psychology is a science that is not a science, and the avoidance of the word "soul" tends to obfuscate this paradoxical status attributed to psychology.

---

[9] "The use of 'psyche' instead of 'soul' is a *new* import into scientific language, an artificial and abstract *technical term* and is clearly inspired by the wish that arose during the 19th century to avoid the traditional word and to cleanse psychology from all the (...) metaphysical, religious overtones and feeling associations and implications of this word (...) By defining psychology with the term psyche you also have *a priori* decided that psychology is limited to meaning a 'part' or one 'aspect' of the human being, in contradistinction to its other parts, such as the body or reason. 'Psyche' integrates the soul into the scientific notion of the natural world at large. (...) the notion of psyche is inalienably tied to the notion of man as its ontic substrate." (Giegerich, *WIS*, pp. 16-17).

Following Jung and Giegerich as well, I am not using "soul" with a spiritual or metaphysical meaning.[10] In the context of my argument, "soul" is used as a synonym for "objective psyche". *It should not be understood as meaning an existing entity or substance.* "Soul" here means *interiority*, the inner psychological dimension of a given phenomenon, and not a subsisting "part" that human being has. "Soul" may thus be defined as the *contra naturam*[11] essence of human being's entire world-relation, the form of his actually lived life as it is seen from the perspective of psychological interiority. From this perspective, interiorization or "soul-making" is the act of considering a given psychic phenomenon exclusively in its own terms, without letting "anything that does not belong to it" come in, thus reaching its psychological objective meaning, its inner symbolic depth, its "soul". Since meaning changes with time, place and culture, with structural shifts in humankind's conscious situation (*CW* 16 §§ 395-396), "soul" is not a static eternal structuring form of human life, but a living historical dynamism. In this intrinsically historical sense one can speak of "soul activity", both on the individual level and on the col-

[10] On the problem and sense of the use of the concept of "soul" in psychological discourse, see Giegerich, *WIS*, pp. 5-87.

[11] Soul as consciousness or mindedness is not simply a natural phenomenon like a tree, a bird or a thunderstorm. It is a new level of life, which pushes off from the natural biological level of life and inaugurates the realm of shared meanings, ideas, fantasies, values, ideals—in a word: culture (see Giegerich, *WIS*, p. 29-44). As such, it can be envisaged as an *opus contra naturam*. It is in this sense that, in order to distinguish a soul event from a natural phenomenon, I use the word "spiritual"—and not in the religious, mystic or metaphysical sense. It only designates the non-natural quality of soul activity. The same is valid to the use of "otherworldliness". It should be noted that if you define "nature" along the lines of Romantic *Naturphilosophie*, this distinction does not properly apply.

lective/cultural level. Thus, "soul activity" refers to the effectively real (*wirklich*) psychological dynamism which produces images, symbols, ideas, thoughts, values, be it individual (such as in a dream or a vision) or cultural (as in a work of art, or in a religious doctrine, for example).

A word about the relation of these two levels—the individual and the cultural—is necessary. The distinction between both levels refers to their different scopes: while a personal dream, for instance, has ordinarily only subjective significance for the individual dreamer, a true work of art, as well as any cultural product, reflects something of the objective state of the collective *ethos*, and thus has a broader and objective significance. If we use the Latin locution "*opus parvum*" to designate the smaller personal-subjective level, we may use its counterpart "*opus magnum*" to designate the broader sphere of culture and historical processes at large (*NB*: both are distinct levels of "soul activity"). Despite this core distinction, sometimes there can be a conjunction of both levels, so that exceptionally a psychic event happening at the level of *opus parvum*, being individual and subjective, may also display something of the psychological dynamism going on at the level of *opus magnum*.

A personalistic psychological approach of any cultural-historical work (such as Freud has adopted in dealing with Leonardo da Vinci's work) loses the "big picture" expressed in that work, inasmuch as it concentrates exclusively on the biographical particularities and accidents of the subject's inner life and explains the work through the personality of its creator. This is no doubt a valid approach. But it misses the whole *opus magnum* dimension of the work. For instance: Picasso's *Guernica* is certainly a very personal work of art, *but* it expresses a vision of the objective situation of culture and humankind in the 20th century at large. *Guernica* is much more than the result of subjective personal psychic mechanisms driving the individual Pablo Picasso. Only an approach focused on the "soul" of the work in its *opus magnum* significance (and not on the personal intricacies of its human *artifex*) can reach its *objective* psychological interiority.

Now, in examining here some of Jung's visions and dreams, I submit that they have the broader reference to soul's *opus magnum* above-mentioned. Jung himself envisaged them in this way.[12] This means that I am not interested in their personal subjective dimension. The personal possibility of a psychotic breakdown, raised by Jung himself at the time of the first visions and dreams (1913), is of no concern to me here. My reflection is not placed in the historiographically problematic area of Jung's personal mental state in 1913-14.

However, I do not follow either the second possibility raised by Jung, which came to be the standard accepted interpretation for his visions and dreams within the Jungian field: their synchronistic, *acausal* correspondence with World War I. *I am not dealing with the notion of synchronicity and its metaphysical aspects.*[13] Jung's interpretation

---

[12] See C.G. Jung. *The Red Book. Liber Novus*. Ed. Sonu Shamdasani. New York/London: W.W. Norton & Co., 2009, pp. 230-231.

[13] A consistent reflection on the relations between synchronicity in Analytical Psychology and modern western culture can be found in Roderick Main. *The Rupture of Time. Synchronicity and Jung's Critique of Modern Western Culture*. Hove/New York: Brunner-Routledge, 2004. On synchronicity interpreted as a form of religious experience, see R. Main. *Revelations of Chance: Synchronicity as Spiritual Experience.* New York: State University of New York Press, 2007. Roderick Main has recently dealt with the secular and religious dimensions of Analytical Psychology (see R. Main. "Secular *and* religious: the intrin-

of his visions and dreams at the time they happened implicitly anticipates the notion of synchronicity, inasmuch as he took them as being *prophetic*. I work here from a different interpretative possibility, opened up by the restricted methodological psychological stance presented above. This choice may be referred to Jung himself: the unconscious "simply creates an image that answers to the conscious situation", and such "an image would be better described as an artist's vision" (*CW* 7 § 289). When a work of art has an anticipatory quality, it does not have to be taken as being literally "prophetic", but more simply as "self-representations of unconscious developments" (*CW* 7 § 216), just like some dreams, with the difference that the developments expressed in a work of art (and, as I claim, in Jung's catastrophic psychic material) belong to the wider horizon of culture, whereas ordinary dreams stay wholly circumscribed to the level of soul's *opus parvum*.

In focusing my reflection at the level of soul's historical *opus magnum*, I attribute a trans-human quality to the psychological dynamism displayed in Jung's visions

---

sic doubleness of analytical psychology and the hegemony of naturalism in the social sciences", in *Journal of Analytical Psychology*, 2013, 58, 366-386). For a masterful disclosure of the roots of Jung's notion of synchronicity in the intellectual tradition, namely as a form of intellectual intuition, see Paul Bishop. *Synchronicity and Intellectual Intuition in Kant, Swedenborg and Jung*. Lewiston/Queenston/Lampeter: Edwin Mellen Press, 2000. Wolfgang Giegerich has discussed the common interpretation of synchronicity in an article published in the *Journal of Analytical Psychology*: see Wolfgang Giegerich. "A serious misunderstanding: synchronicity and the generation of meaning", in *Journal of Analytical Psychology*, 2012, 57, 500-511; see also Warren Colman's reply to Giegerich in the same issue: W. Colman. "Reply to Wolfgang Giegerich's 'A serious misunderstanding: synchronicity and the generation of meaning'", in *Journal of Analytical Psychology*, 2012, 57, 512-516.

and dreams. This should not be understood as some mysterious or religious dimension of the psychic material. It simply means that the immanent *telos* (goal or aim) of soul activity is its own self-actualization, *regardless of the human subject's interests or concerns*. As a "dark urge" or "unclear impulse", a "longing and telos", soul activity has a fundamental process character, which aims at the completion of its "full reality in the empirical world and real life".[14] In this very particular sense, a psychologically creative individual is able to follow soul's *telos* regardless of his/her own interests, just for the sake of the "logos of the soul".

Jung certainly had that capability. As is well known, Jung stated that all his work came from the fantasies and dreams he had during his "confrontation with the unconscious", the *prima materia* which compelled him to work upon it, and which he compares to a "stream of lava". He saw his Analytical Psychology as "a more or less successful endeavor to incorporate this incandescent matter into the contemporary picture of the world".[15] We could say, drawing on Jung's thought about the dream being its own interpretation, that this "incandescent matter" is already a self-interpretation of "the contemporary picture of the world", it *is* this picture (obviously only to a certain extent), although, as Jung said, "at first only in the form of emotions and images".[16]

Within Jung's "stream of lava", there are some particular images, gushing forth at an early moment of his crea-

---

[14] Giegerich, *WIS*, p. 41 and 43.
[15] Jung, *MDR*, p. 199.
[16] Jung, *MDR*, p. 192.

tive founding experience, which call our attention due to their extremely dark content: the impressive twice repeated catastrophic vision he had at the end of 1913, as well as the thrice repeated dream of a similar nature he had in the first half of 1914. This apocalyptic initial material is akin to the tragic dimension of the 20th century, so that Jung's catastrophic vision and dreams could be understood as fateful psychological events, arguably having some kinship (regarding their common inner logic) to fateful contemporary historical events. Thus all of them—the psychological as well as the historical events—manifest some relation to soul's *opus magnum*.

The catastrophic content reappears at the very end of Jung's life (and work), in 1961, in the context of a truly archetypal experience—his imminent death—, again in the form of a vision. We have only an extremely brief allusion to this last vision, made by Marie-Louise von Franz, and this determines the narrow limit within which we can explore it. However, its catastrophic content is beyond any doubt, and one can see that it is significantly different from the psychic material of 1913-1914. My working hypothesis is that this last vision could be considered as the psychological closure of that same soul experience on which Analytical Psychology is grounded, and at the same time the opening—or anticipation—of a radically new situation, to which it is not fitted anymore. Therefore one could envision Jung's work as framed and deeply determined by a psychological catastrophe, from its beginning to its end. And I shall argue that this catastrophe is not only Jung's, but, on the contrary, refers to the psychological configuration of the modern form of consciousness, a configuration which has been fully realized or has completely exteriorized itself in history during the 20th century. This is what I intend to show in what follows.

The Visions and Dreams of 1913-1914

It may be interesting to note that "catastrophe" comes from the Greek *katastrophé*, which means a sudden end, an overturning (*katastrophé* is composed of *kata*, "down", and *strophein*, "turn", so that literally taken a catastrophe is a "turning down"). The word has its origins in Ancient Greek tragedy: it designated the moment in which events turned against the main character, in a movement executed by the whole chorus in the theater. It was a fateful turning point. Catastrophe thus, according to Merriam-Webster, is "a momentous tragic event ranging from extreme misfortune to utter overthrow or ruin".[17]

Jung's experience in 1913-1914, having at its center the apocalyptic vision, fulfills the original meaning of *katastrophé*, not only in the personal sphere, but also in the psychological structure of the soul event *falling upon* him, which expresses itself in his feeling of falling down—we must only remember the moment, in the Advent of 1913 (December 12), when Jung finally gives up and lets himself *drop*, and says: "Suddenly it was as though the ground literally gave way beneath my feet, and I plunged down in dark depths".[18] This is surely the psychic experience of *katastrophé*, "turning down".

---

[17] Merriam-Webster Online Dictionary, http://www.merriam-webster.com/dictionary/catastrophe, accessed 21 May 2020.
[18] Jung, *MDR*, p. 179.

Jung describes the whole catastrophe in very dramatic terms. I will follow here step by step the sequence of the narrative presented in *Memories, Dreams, Reflections*.[19]

> Toward the autumn of 1913 the pressure which I had felt was in *me* seemed to be moving outward, as though there were something in the air. The atmosphere actually seemed to me darker than it had been. It was as though the sense of oppression no longer sprang exclusively from a psychic situation, but from concrete reality. This feeling grew more and more intense. (*MDR*, p. 175)

Jung feels a movement from an exclusively inward location ("in *me*") to an outward emplacement ("as though there were something in the air"). He interprets this movement as a convergence of a merely subjective "psychic situation" and positive-factual objective "concrete reality". Nonetheless, one can also concentrate exclusively on the contents of the whole situation and think it through, taking its two sides ("psychic situation" and "concrete reality") *psychologically*, and leave aside the blinding fascination of the possible positive-factual synchronistic coincidence. In this way, from the outset "concrete reality" is taken as indicating the activity of the *objective psyche*, a self-presentation of soul's dynamism, and can thus be interiorized. Let us remember the methodological rule: neither the individual "in here", nor the world "out there", but soul itself. This is the specific condition for reaching (or producing) the psychological dimension, understood as the in-

---

[19] Jung, *MDR*, pp. 175-176. See also Jung, *The Red Book*, pp. 230-235 [Liber Primus folios i(v) to ii(v)]; and the introductory seminar on Analytical Psychology: C.G. Jung. *Analytical Psychology. Notes of the Seminar Given in 1925.* Ed. William McGuire. Princeton: Princeton University Press, 1989, pp. 41-44.

depth interiority of a given phenomenon. From this perspective, the psychic atmosphere indicates an *extra*-ordinary or non-ordinary circumstance. There is a transition going on. Jung is crossing a threshold: from ordinary subjective perspective ("the pressure which I had felt was in *me*") to an uncanny perspective (a darker atmosphere, "concrete reality", "as though the sense of oppression no longer sprang exclusively from a psychic situation"). This transition of perspective is also signaled in that fateful moment of his crisis when he feels he is "plunging down into dark depths".

The vision and the three dreams that subsequently follow confirm this transition to an objective, impersonal level.

> In October [1913], while I was alone on a journey, I was suddenly seized by an overpowering vision: I saw a monstrous flood covering all the northern and low-lying lands between the North Sea and the Alps. When it came up to Switzerland I saw that the mountains grew higher and higher to protect our country. I realized that a frightful catastrophe was in progress. I saw the mighty yellow waves, the floating rubble of civilization, and the drowned bodies of uncounted thousands. Then the whole sea turned to blood. This vision lasted about one hour. I was perplexed and nauseated, and ashamed of my weakness. (*MDR*, p. 175)

A brutal upheaval destroys the north European region: civilization is reduced to rubble, a portion of mankind is wiped out. On the semantic level, the catastrophe is imaged as a *monstrous flood*—which means that it is not the result of human activity, or rather that it does not spring from the human realm. Just like the Biblical deluge, it comes from some trans-human source, which is oriented to and affects mainly the human realm. Following this analogy, Switzerland protected by the mountains may be functionally compared, to a certain extent, to Noah's ark: something is preserved from the catastrophic destruction. There is a remainder of the old order: Switzerland is safely protected (through the rising mountains) from the "frightful catastrophe [that] was in progress".[20] I will return to this detail. For now, it should be noted that both the destructive flood *and* the protective barrier against it belong equally to the soul activity going on and pictorially represented in the vision.

> Two weeks passed; then the vision recurred, under the same conditions, even more vividly than before, and the blood was more emphasized. An inner voice spoke. "Look at it well; it is wholly real and it will be so. You cannot doubt it". (*MDR*, p. 175)

The water turns into blood. This is not to be taken as a causal-natural result of the "drowned bodies of uncounted thousands": firstly, because drowning does not imply bleeding; secondly, because even if it did, the blood of uncounted thousands would not suffice to turn *the whole sea* into blood. No. The vision presents a strange transformation from water to blood, comparable to the transubstantiation of wine into blood in the Eucharist. There is an uncanny transformation taking place, a non-natural event—a soul event. And the reality of the mysterious transformation as well as of the whole soul process is emphasized, not necessarily as a (possible) synchronistic premonition of the brutal posi-

[20] By the way, what an interesting and suggestive double sense in the English translation here! The German original has "Eine schreckliche Katastrophe spielte sich ab", which could also be freely translated as "a frightful catastrophe was happening".

tive-factual war that soon was going to follow externally (this is alien to the image, it comes from outside as an *a posteriori* conjectural interpretation): sticking firmly to the image, and to the methodological stance of a discipline of interiority, it is *the vision itself* that is wholly real and will be so. Soul activity reinforces by means of the inner voice its own reality, its objectivity—in the sense of "objective psyche".

> That winter someone asked me what I thought were the political prospects of the world in the near future. I replied that I had no thoughts on the matter, but that I saw rivers of blood.
> I asked myself whether these visions pointed to a revolution, but could not imagine anything of the sort. And so I drew the conclusion that they had to do with me myself, and decided that I was menaced by a psychosis. The idea of war did not occur to me at all. (*MDR*, pp. 175-176)

Jung at first sees only two possible alternatives: either a personal subjective pathology (psychosis), or an external positive-factual event (revolution, war). And I think one should not simply dismiss these possibilities. It is plausible to think that there was a real risk of a psychotic breakdown. Were the circumstances different, leading to a failure in the elaboration of his dramatic crisis, a psychosis could have ensued—Jung certainly was well acquainted with this possibility as a psychiatrist at the Burghölzli. On the other hand, World War I was indeed a bloody human catastrophe, a real positive-factual revolution, signaling the end of a phase of modern history and the beginning of the catastrophic 20th century. However, a rigorously psychological approach takes the vision *as vision*, that is, as a psychic event on its own, regardless of its possible impact on the individual's psychic equilibrium or its correspondence with an external event. Only by following this approach can we try to reflect the soul truth displayed in the vision.

The primordial act of soul activity, through and in which soul creates itself anew, or creates a new form of consciousness, is the negation of a previous form, from which it pushes off. This "pushing off" is represented as killing, destruction, catastrophe, death. So the monstrous destructive flood could, in these terms, be seen as displaying the negating activity of soul, which is exerted on "civilization" and "humankind". Accepting that civilization and human form of existence are expressions of soul activity, it becomes clear that in Jung's vision soul is negating *itself*, it is destroying an accomplished level of itself. However, the preservation of Switzerland from the negation/destruction shows that in Jung's vision the negation is countered by a conservative movement of soul itself. This means that the negation is not absolute, the transformation portrayed is not fully accomplished, since there is a remainder of the old configuration, preserved from the transformative drive.

If we move now to the thrice repeated dream, we will find the same catastrophic motif (though with a different symbolization), displaying both the self-negation going on and the unfolding of the resistance that soul is opposing to itself, disclosing its goal.

> Soon afterward, in the spring and early summer of 1914, I had a thrice-repeated dream that in the middle of summer an Arctic cold wave descended and froze the land to ice. I saw, for example, the whole of Lorraine and its canals frozen and the entire region totally deserted by human beings. All living green things were killed by frost. This dream came in April and May, and for the last time in June, 1914. (*MDR*, p. 176)

Envisaging the dreams as an expression of the same soul process portrayed in the catastrophic vision, we can say that the prime matter suffers a transformation: from the heat of a sea of blood to the frost of an Arctic cold. The change from the blood-heat of recently destroyed life in the vision to the cold of frozen death in the dreams is indicative of a deepening of soul's "deadly" negating activity. Empirically, the more one moves away from natural life, often the colder it gets (extreme heat and extreme cold are incompatible with biological life as we know it). Psychologically envisaged, the "icy-cold" character of soul activity indicates the special active relation of soul and death.[21] We can even say that "soul" is the interiorization of death into life, a movement that creates consciousness (and *is* consciousness itself) and opens up the specifically human form of existence.

The transformation of consciousness through the negation of a previous stage of itself is the psychological form of death. But this death "could in no way have been that innocent death that merely *happens* to a living being as a natural life event to be passively endured. No, it must be death in the active sense, as the unnatural, outrageous, deliberate act of killing".[22] In the vision, the unnatural quality of the death is indicated by the transmutation of the deadly sea into blood; in the dreams, by the uncanny detail that frost occurs in the middle of summer. There is clearly something out of the natural order, extra-ordinary.

---

[21] On this topic, see E. Herzog. *Psyche and Death. Death-Demons in Folklore, Myths and Modern Dreams*. Woodstock: Spring Publications, 1983.

[22] Giegerich, *CEP III*, p. 215.

The frozen death of the dreams kills all living green things, the green life. It reaches beyond the animal/human level (blood organisms), and affects the first stage of life: vegetation. The landscape is totally inhospitable to human beings, indicating the exclusion of the human point of view.

> In the third dream frightful cold had again descended from out of the cosmos. This dream, however, had an unexpected end. There stood a leaf-bearing tree, but without fruit (my tree of life, I thought), whose leaves had been transformed by the effects of the frost into sweet grapes full of healing juices. I plucked the grapes and gave them to a large, waiting crowd. (*MDR*, p. 176)

Now, here the catastrophe acquires a cosmic dimension, and this stresses its otherworldly, trans-human nature. This expansion of the frame, so to speak, is signified by the appearance of the leaf-bearing tree: the deepening of the frozen death makes the source of life appear. And it is a strange tree, which endures frost, and thus does not belong to the same level of the previously destroyed "living green things". It is a supernatural tree, uncanny, the "tree of life", which has a different relation to "death": unlike the individual natural trees, which were simply destroyed, this "tree of life" has a deep dialectical relation to "frozen death". If "soul" is "death" interiorized into "life", so that "ensouled life" is plainly consciousness (or psychological life), then we can understand the identity of "frost" and "tree of life" as an expression of the dynamism of consciousness.

That the tree of life *is* dialectically the frost itself becomes patent in its fruits. For these grapes are no ordinary, natural fruits: frost turned the green leaves into sweet grapes, which is impossible on the naturalistic dimension.

They resulted from a different kind of transformation. And therefore the grapes also are strange: not only are they frost itself in the form of transformed leaves, but they are full of "*healing juices*"—which means that frost is healing. Just as in the Bible Yahweh formed mankind (*homo*) from the dust of the ground (*humus*) by breathing the breath of spiritual life (the divine *pneuma*, divine life) into the nostrils of Adam (*adâm* comes from *adamá*, the soil), thus transmitting Himself to the new human form, frost in the dream transmits itself as healing juices in the new form of grapes.

Whilst it is life-destroying on the naturalistic level, the dream's frost (soul's icy-coldness) is life-giving on the spiritual level. This means that the grapes are not fit to nurture or give sensorial pleasure in the biological, bodily sense: they are meant to *heal* the spirit. They have a psychological ("*spiritual*") meaning. Their healing juices make them analogous to the Eucharistic *bread and wine* (taken in their symbolic/psychological signification). The grapes are definitely not ordinary grapes, but a *healing substance*. As such, they come from a transformation involving sacrificial death: just like Christ's body and blood. Consequently, we are faced here with a kind of communion: the self-transformation of soul is extended, through the giving of the grapes, to "a large, waiting crowd".

Jung only plucks and gives the grapes: he is not their source, which is the frost. So, in the dream Jung acts in a way similar to the priest in the Catholic Mass: he is only an instrument to the transformation/transubstantiation, whose real cause is soul activity. We can further explore this analogy: in the Mass—and in the dream—the "terrors of death are an indispensable condition for the transformation", which is "in the first place a bringing to life of substances which are in themselves lifeless, and, in the second, a substantial alteration of them, a spiritualization, in accordance with the ancient conception of *pneuma* as a subtle material entity" (*CW* 11 § 338). And "man, too, by his devotion and self-sacrifice as a ministering instrument, is included in the mysterious process" (*CW* 11 § 338). The destructive-creative activity of soul, imaged as frost, gives birth to (or presents itself as) a new level of spiritual life (*as* healing juice to humankind) through killing the naturalistic level of conscious perception (the natural green life). This, I claim, would be the resumed soul truth imagistically presented in the dream—and the core of the entire soul catastrophe also (partly) represented in the vision.

But we should also stress here the difference between Jung's soul event and the Christian Mass. There's no mention of "God", no explicit religious feeling associated with the vision and the dreams. The uncanny aspect of the "catastrophe in progress" does not have a religious content. It only points to the (by definition) unnatural form of soul activity. And finally, the difference can be made explicit by our focusing on one element of the dream image: Jung himself. It is not a priest who is *causa ministerialis* in the dream, but a man whose life was (and would continue to be from then on) deeply identified with *psychology*, the very same man who "*had a real Notion or Concept of 'soul'* ".[23] This notion seized Jung, imposed itself on him—remember the inner voice in the vision: "Look at it well; it is wholly real and it will be so. You cannot doubt it". So, the human sacrifice in the vision and the turning down—*katastrophé*—

[23] Wolfgang Giegerich. *The Soul's Logical Life*. Frankfurt am Main: Peter Lang, 3rd edition, 2001, p. 41.

in the vision and dreams represent soul transmitting itself in the new form of *psychology*, and not of *religion*. Jung's psychology sublates religion. Accordingly, Jung's understanding of his work as "a more or less successful endeavor to incorporate this incandescent [and, dialectically, frozen] matter into the contemporary picture of the world" is perfectly grounded in the third dream: he would indeed pluck the soul's grapes and offer them to a vast crowd. His life's work would really be an event rooted in that transformation and in the real objective notion of soul. As such, his was truly a catastrophic psychology.

On the other hand, as pointed out above, the "catastrophe in progress" was not absolute. Soul preserves "Switzerland" from its destructive-negating activity in the vision. Something of its initial status is conserved, a self-conservation takes place. If now we merge "Switzerland" with "Jung plucking and giving the grapes", the result is that his psychology, being an expression of its grounding soul event and *wholly* committed to it (as this event effectively happened to him), *necessarily would present a conservative thrust*. Jung acknowledges his personal conservatism[24], but the conservatism we can easily find in the very theoretical structure of his thought should not be attributed merely to his personal inclinations, *but to his psychology's founding soul event itself*. Jung explicitly defends his kind

[24] See Jung, *MDR*, p. 358. Jay Sherry (*Carl Gustav Jung: Avant-Garde Conservative*. New York: Palgrave Macmillan, 2010) explores Jung's relations to the conflicts and problems of modernity, and relativizes the simple opposition between conservatism and modernity by showing how Jung's conservative profile can be seen as a form of modern (or "avant-garde") stance. This particular stance is presented in "The Spiritual Problem of Modern Man" (see CW 10 §§ 152-154). Evidently, Jung's "modern man" is a description of his own stance.

of "reforming conservatism" in the broader frame of cultural-historical life.[25]

In being absolutely true to his catastrophic founding vision and dreams of 1913-1914, Jung has consciously proposed in his psychology a "reform by retrogression".[26] A certain conception of humankind and civilization (in continuity with the classical and Christian traditions) was preserved and spared from negation in that founding soul event. "Man" is the highest value in this conception. Furthermore, Jung's "psychology with soul" is, in a deep sense, *anthropo-logically biased*[27]—being thus structurally *modern.* In this sense, Jung's catastrophic psychology is simultaneously anti-catastrophic: being fundamentally soul based, it expresses the (then still) *historically* unresolved particular opposition of soul to itself. "Switzerland", as a momentary and contemporary "Noah's ark", was not yet dissolved by the power of the negative.

I think this accounts for the ambiguity we can detect in Jung's conservative project (and also in a vast portion of his followers, of those who waited for and received the "healing grapes"): as the radical transformation going on was not absolute, the destruction of the old forms also could not be complete. And so "psychology" in Jung could not be radically separated from "anthropology" and from "religion" (inasmuch as the notions of "Man" and "God", struc-

---

[25] See Jung, *MDR*, pp. 235-237.

[26] In the German original the expression used is "Verbesserungen nach rückwärts"; "Verbesserung" is not exactly "reform", but "improvement".

[27] See M.H. Barreto. "God, Man and Evil in Jung's Thought. Complementary Remarks to Wolfgang Giegerich's Critique", in *Spring: a Journal of Archetype and Culture* (New Orleans, vol. 84, Fall 2010, p. 107-141).

turing the old level of consciousness, presumably were preserved from the destruction/sublation in the spared region of "Switzerland").

> At the end of July 1914 I was invited by the British Medical Association to deliver a lecture, "On the Importance of the Unconscious in Psychopathology", at a congress in Aberdeen. I was prepared for something to happen, for such visions and dreams are fateful. In my state of mind just then, with the fears that were pursuing me, it seemed fateful to me that I should have to talk on the importance of the unconscious at such a time!
> On August 1 the world war broke out. Now my task was clear: I had to try to understand what had happened and to what extent my own experience coincided with that of mankind in general. Therefore my first obligation was to probe the depths of my own psyche. I made a beginning by writing down the fantasies which had come to me during my building game. This work took precedence over everything else. (*MDR*, p. 176)

Until the irruption of the world war, Jung was living the catastrophe on a subjective level (the one in which he thought there was a risk of psychosis). But then the second possibility considered by Jung (war, revolution) became concrete. Although he does not consider the third alternative explicitly, we can say that it was immersed, buried, implicit in the way he tried to understand the inner and outer events. And the risk of a personalistic reduction of the whole experience ("*my* tree of life, I thought") is countered by his considering that his experience coincided "with that of mankind in general". Jung understood there to be an objective level of the process he was living, and saw that the problem was one of the times—in the same way as he realized that his *personal* identification with the Faustian issue was a misunderstanding, because "Goethe's strange heroic myth was a collective experience".[28]

This psychological constellation was effective in 1913-1914. But the "psychic atmosphere" would change, and the catastrophe was to have a further development.

The Last Vision, 1961

The experience of world wars in the 20th century exerted a traumatic and deep impact on European consciousness and affected Jung as well. After the Second World War, he wrote to Esther Harding: "Switzerland has become an island of dreams amidst ruins and putrefaction. Europe is a rotting carcass".[29] Jung's engagement with the healing of civilization prevailed in the last decades of his life. True to Analytical Psychology's founding visions and dreams, he tried to find a way to preserve the continuity of culture. He believed that the cure for the split in modern consciousness was buried in the Christian roots of Western civilization, and so he dedicated all his efforts to "the psychological reinvigoration of Christianity".[30] There it is: a "reform by retrogression".

However, to Jung the conscious confrontation of "the actual existing man" with "his own demons" seemed "to be a losing fight", at least for the time being.[31] To such confrontation Analytical Psychology was devised. No won-

---

[28] Jung, *MDR*, p. 234.

[29] July 8, 1947, quoted in Sonu Shamdasani. *Jung and the Making of Modern Psychology. The Dream of a Science*. Cambridge: Cambridge University Press, 2003, p. 349.

[30] Shamdasani, *Jung and the Making of Modern Psychology*, p. 350

[31] See Shamdasani, *Jung and the Making of Modern Psychology*, p. 349.

der, then, that Jung's pessimism concerning the fate of the world would be extended to his own work. At the end of his life he experienced a strong feeling of failure, and expressed this in a letter to Eugene Rolfe, dated November 13, 1960:

> I had to understand, that I was unable to make people see, what I am after. I am practically alone… I have failed in my foremost task, to open people's eyes to the fact, that man has a soul and there is a buried treasure in the field and that our religion and philosophy are in a lamentable state. Why indeed should I continue to exist?[32]

If we leave aside the personal inflated identification of Jung with his projected cultural task for psychology, an inflation envisaged by Michael Fordham as a "delusion of being a world savior",[33] the failure felt by Jung is of depth psychology itself as a source of collective compensation for "what was lacking in the West".[34] Shamdasani comments:

> Judging by these late letters, in Jung's own estimation, complex psychology—and psychology as a whole—had failed to make sufficient social impact, and hence failed to provide adequate antidotes to the "fathers and mothers of all terrors".[35]

Jung believed that psychology should provide the medicine for the dilacerations in modern consciousness (see the "healing grapes" of the 1914 dream). Arguably the most crystal clear testimonies of his concern with the catastrophic

---

[32] Quoted in Shamdasani, *Jung and the Making of Modern Psychology*, p. 351.
[33] Quoted in Shamdasani, *Jung and the Making of Modern Psychology*, p. 351.
[34] Shamdasani, *Jung and the Making of Modern Psychology*, p. 351.
[35] Shamdasani, *Jung and the Making of Modern Psychology*, p. 352.

possibilities present in the unfolding of contemporary history are his later essays *The Undiscovered Self (Present and Future)* (1957) and *Flying Saucers: A Modern Myth* (1958). In them one can find his speculations about the ways of protecting and healing modern humankind from the disintegrating forces that would fatefully change its cultural form.

The failure of psychology in this inflated (and thus unrealistic) projected task of rescuing a lost balance in the wider scale of the world is a historical fact. This cultural project became obsolete in the face of the structural and radical changes in the world. Depth psychology was devised for a specific modern form of being-in-the-world, which was superseded by another form, not anymore represented by "depth", "interiority" or "soul" (in Jung's sense). This new situation was painfully experienced by Jung, and it can be read in the impressive final visions which he had in 1961.

According to the testimony of Marie-Louise von Franz, recorded in the documentary *Matter of Heart*, when she saw Jung last he had a vision (while she was with him), and said: "I see enormous stretches devastated, enormous stretches of the earth, but thank God it's not the whole planet". Here the catastrophe is not portrayed anymore as restricted to a particular region of the Earth: it has become planetary, globalized, so to speak. But, just as in the vision of 1913 Switzerland was protected by the rising mountains from the monstrous flood, here too some portion of the planet is still preserved. Thus, the moment of the soul process displayed in this penultimate vision has still some inner reservation, it is still not absolute negation. This could further an optimistic hope to an ego-psychologically oriented consciousness, a hope related to its self-preservation.

However, immediately before his death Jung had another catastrophic vision whose content was "the last fifty years of humanity". Notes were taken by one of his daughters, with some remarks about the final catastrophe being ahead. There is no mention of a remainder preserved from the destruction. The final catastrophe ahead seems to be absolute. Therefore, this last vision is more radical: it depicts humanity as on the eve of its *total* extinction. And this means that the soul truth symbolically articulated in the catastrophic vision (and, according to my working hypothesis, in Jung's psychology as such) will finally be absolutely realized. More than just a psychic event announcing the literal death of the individual Carl Gustav Jung, the vision anticipates the coming logical death of his psychology's human presuppositions, within "fifty years". The soul experience of which it is the "more or less successful" expression comes to its logical conclusion. In Jung's final vision, soul in advance sings the requiem for Analytical Psychology, which is its own (soul's) requiem—at least in the form it takes in the conservative "reform by retrogression" embodied in Jung's psychology of the unconscious.

To avoid any misunderstanding, I must now make a clear remark: when I use the concept of "humankind" in the interpretation of Jung's catastrophic psychic material, I have in mind only a very restricted, particular sense of this notion, namely one embodied in the *modern anthropocentric form of humanism*, with its classical and Christian roots. It is to *this* particular sense of "humankind" that Jung's psychology is addressed. It is *this* notion that it partly expresses. So, if the "last fifty years of humanity" in Jung's final vision on his death-bed imagistically displays the extinction of human presence in the world, its radical dehumanization, then from the perspective of psychology as a discipline of interiority this should only be interpreted as the overcoming of a specific *notion of humanity*, the one for which Analytical Psychology was devised.

Marie-Louise von Franz interprets the vision in a prophetic-apocalyptic perspective, as referring to the literal destruction of humankind:

> I don't want to speak much about it. (…) One's whole feeling revolts against this idea. But since I have those notes in the drawer I don't allow myself to be too optimistic. I think, well, we have always had wars and enormous catastrophes, and I have no more personal fears much about that (…). But the beauty of all life, and to think of the billions and billions and billions of years that took evolution to build up the plants and the animals, and the whole beauty of nature, and that man would go out of sheer shallow foolishness and destroy it all, I mean that all life might go from the planet. And we don't know—on Mars and Venus there is no life—we don't know if there is any life experiment elsewhere in the galaxies. And we go and destroy this. I think it's so abominable. I try to pray that it may not happen—that a miracle happens. (…) Because if you think of *Answer to Job*, if man would wrestle with God, if man would tell God that He shouldn't do it, if we would reflect more… That's why reflection comes in. Jung never thought that we might do better than just possibly sneak around the corner, with not too big a catastrophe. (…) I think that if not more people try to reflect and take back their projections, and take the opposites within themselves, there will be a total destruction. (Marie-Louise von Franz, transcribed from the interview in *Matter of Heart*)

Von Franz's interpretation could invoke the precedent of Jung himself, who interpreted the vision of destruction he had in 1913 as an announcement of the coming world war. And, as a matter of fact, this hypothesis is not negligible: the possibility of a drastic collapse of humanity cannot be dismissed anymore as being simply a paranoid delusion. But to the methodological and self-definitional stance of psychology as the discipline of interiority, this hypothesis is neither here nor there, for the *sole* interest of this specific psychological stance is precisely in the *inner psychological articulation of the image, its logical life.*

Nevertheless, one can indicate an empirical correspondent to the soul truth expressed in Jung's final vision. Here I will focus on a telling moment of von Franz's interview:

> [Young people seem today to be] giving up and running away into a fantasy world. When you study science fiction, you see there is always the fantasy of escaping to some other planet and beginning anew again, which means give up the battle on this earth. Consider it hopeless and give up. I think one shouldn't give up (Marie-Louise von Franz, transcribed from the interview in *Matter of Heart*).

But isn't this precisely what happens in medial modernity, the new form of living in a virtual space? "This earth", or the quality of realness or givenness of "this earth", is replaced by the technologically fabricated conditions of existence. "Fantasy" has prevailed. The active giving up of "this earth" has posited a new form of world and of being-in-the-world. The new forms of subjectivity emerging from the radically different techno-environment that molds our contemporary world do not correspond to the analytical (or psychoanalytical) understanding of human being.

In Jung's last vision, humanity is *sacrificed*. The sacrificial act requires a *complete* destruction of the gift to be sacrificed:

> The gift always carries with it a personal intention, for the mere giving of it is not a sacrifice. It only becomes a sacrifice if I give up the implied intention of receiving something in return. If it is to be a true sacrifice, the gift must be given as if it were being destroyed. Only then it is possible for the egoistic claim to be given up. (...) Consequently, all absolute giving, a giving which is a total loss from the start, is a self-sacrifice. Ordinary giving for which no return is received is felt as a loss; but a sacrifice is meant to be like a loss, so that one may be sure that the egoistic claim no longer exists. Therefore the gift should be given as if it were being destroyed. (CW 11 § 390)
> Every sacrifice is therefore, to a greater or lesser degree, a self-sacrifice. (...) If it is of great value to me and touches my most personal feelings, I can be sure that in giving up my egoistic claim I shall challenge my ego personality to revolt (CW 11 § 397).

Jung's reflections on absolute giving, and on sacrifice as total destruction (of the offering) is in blatant contrast with von Franz's desperate hope of stopping the (literal) destruction by means of struggling with God as Job did (did he?), which is also to say, by means of individual reflection, taking back the projections, taking the opposites within oneself. Von Franz sees the (*visionary idea* of) destruction of humankind and the planet as an act of God, and revolts against this. She is not in the same position as Job at the end of his experience: she is in Job's initial position, arguing with God, previous to the theophany which transforms Job's consciousness. She insists on the "egoistic claim", for "one's whole feeling *revolts* against this idea", as she states in the interview in *Matter of Heart*. By so doing, she does not accomplish the *total sacrifice* in Jung's terms. And thus she stands *against* the vision, interpreting it literally.

If the essence of a particular historical *human* mode of being-in-the-world is logically sacrificed and/or negated, this only means that, as Günther Anders has seen long ago,[36] humankind has itself become antiquated as the fundamental agent and addressee of the logic of the world (soul's *opus magnum*), not necessarily that the human species is on the verge of its literal extinction. This, in the last analysis, is what Jung's final vision presents, from a strictly psychological perspective: the humanistic age is over.[37]

The destruction of humankind in Jung's last vision means very simply that soul negates the last sacred and highest Western value—the idea of human dignity, of "man as such" as the ultimate humanistic goal of civilization. This value was preserved from destruction (negation) in the vision of 1913, through the rising mountains that protected Switzerland. Logically, the idea of human dignity (transposed to the declaration of human rights) requires the intactness of the person, which includes "the necessity to protect the intact physical existence (i.e., life) of each empirical person".[38] The imaginal way of representing this final and absolute negation is, thus, the absolute destruction of humankind, without remainders. This is what arguably is im-

---

[36] See Günther Anders. *Die Antiquiertheit des Menschen. Über die Seele im Zeitalter der zweiten industriellen Revolution.* München: C. H. Beck, 1956.

[37] See Umberto Galimberti's description of the "new vices" that allow us to have a glimpse of the essence of the new form of being-in-the-world prevalent in medial modernity (U. Galimberti. *Os Vícios Capitais e os Novos Vícios*. São Paulo: Paulus, 2003).

[38] Giegerich, *CEP III*, p. 424

plied in "the last fifty years of mankind". It corresponds to the deep objective truth of Western contemporary society in the Age of Technique.

What comes after the symbolic "destruction of humankind" on the logical level is what can be designated as the post-modern or, using a newly widespread expression, *post-human* logical status of consciousness. This form can be grasped through the perception that our world is not *really, truly* organized having as its goal concrete human benefits, but it is the other way around: concrete human beings serve the goals of the great systems of technology and economics, as replaceable parts in the process of those objective systems. In face of the total logical sublatedness of the human position in this same world, we are again living within the logic of human sacrifice which prevailed in many ancient cultures, with the difference that this time the sacrifice is not performed only on an individual victim, and on a special occasion, but absolutely realized all the time and on all of us. It is the perfect sacrifice. This, I submit, is the soul meaning of "the final catastrophe" seen by Jung on his death-bed, which is quite different from the (possible) positive-factual destruction of the human species, of *homo sapiens*. Correlative of the full accomplishment of the psychological form of consciousness proposed in Jung's life experience, the catastrophe implies the logical end of his psychology of the unconscious. For this psychology soul sings its requiem through Jung's final vision, as a way of saying of its own *opus*: *Consummatum est.*[39]

---

[39] This means only that the humanistic ideals which informed Analytical Psychology—think of the "confrontation with the unconscious" as a modern version of Socrates's "know thyself", and the "process of individuation" as a modern version of Pindar's "become such as you are,

having learned what that is"—are not anymore representative of the objective logic of the world. In this specific sense they are "logically obsolete". Concerning the empirical perspectives of Jungian analysis after the "final catastrophe", I agree with Giegerich's standpoint: though it is thinkable that Jungian analysis is nearing its end, other possibilities are: 1) its metamorphosis into pop psychology (which has already been accomplished to a good extent), 2) its genuine persistence as a way of practicing the original goals of self-knowledge and individuation as conceived by Jung (a marginal form of living, with regards to the "general trend of society away from analysis"). Giegerich reminds us that the shrinking of Jungian analysis' presence in society could "represent a new chance for it, the chance to become aware of what is really significant". (in Robert and Janis Henderson. *Living with Jung. "Enterviews" with Jungian Analysts. Volume 3.* New Orleans: Spring Journal Books, 2010, p. 293).

Chapter 2
The End of Man in the Modern Form of Consciousness

To summarize in a nutshell the thesis presented in the previous chapter, I submit that Jung's catastrophic visions display the psychological framework within which his psychological project was devised, even as they convey the purpose and conditions of validity of the latter. I maintain that Jung's psychology is meant to address a very specific modern human form of being-in-the-world, symbolized in the 1913 vision by the remnant of humanity spared from the catastrophe through the protective mountain barriers surrounding Switzerland, and that the final catastrophe portrayed in the last vision of 1961 completely destroys this circumscribed remnant of the modern notion of "Man", so that Jung's psychological project finds its *logical* end (not necessarily the end of its empirical presence in the cultural landscape of the contemporary world).

I would like to provide a further ground to the conclusions reached in my interpretation, through a philosophical approach, both phenomenological and historical. Basically, as a counterpoint to the specific notion of "Man" which is a presupposition of Analytical Psychology (and whose logical destruction is depicted in Jung's visionary "final catastrophe"), I will present the new form that replaces this notion after its logical obsolescence, a form which is correlative of the new mode of being-in-the-world prevalent after the radical changes brought about in humankind's way of life by the Industrial Revolution. This form is that of *Mass Man*. Since its inception, it has co-existed with the previous form, representative of Western humanism especially in its anthropocentric version. The twilight of this anthropocentric humanism is correlative of the full triumph in culture of Mass Man. This triumph reaches its most recent contours in medial modernity, in which the form of being-in-the-world is defined by the essential and irrevocable merger of mass-minded Man and the technological-cybernetic apparatus which molds the actual environment inside which we all live in the Age of Technique. This corresponds to the last phase in the relations of "human" and "machine" as established in the logic of the Industrial Revolution, the same logic which is responsible for the effective *massification* (*Vermassung*), the revolutionary restructuring of humankind as a mass. In the early stages of this process, human beings were integrated into the technical-mechanical productive environment as distinct agents performing specific actions in the production system (much like some horses are coupled to a chariot to make it move). The system could engulf and even seriously threaten the humanity of the agents (see Charles Chaplin's *Modern Times*), but there was still a fundamental difference between human agent and technical environment. In the current advanced phase, by contrast, not only technology invades and encompasses *all* of the human spheres of life, but it also invades very literally the inner human constitution (as is most evident in the interventions made possible by nanotechnologies), so that the concept of "man-machine" (La Méttrie) turns out to be the real truth of the human condition in the Age of Technique. One cannot anymore distinguish between man and machine. As the horses have been sublated into automobile engines as "horsepower", rendering animal traction obsolete, so human capacities are sublated into the technical environment, rendering the notion of "human *nature*" (or *essence*) obsolete.

After presenting the typical features of Mass Man/mass-mindedness, I will expose its source in the logical constitution of modern consciousness, showing how it both furthers early modern humanism and the logical condition of its destruction and/or obsolescence.

Mass Man, Mass-mindedness: a Brief Phenomenological Description

Mass Man is a product and an expression of modernity. The coming of a mass age, with the correlative rise of the Mass Man, had already been predicted early in the 19th century by scholars and statesmen who could see and anticipate the consequences of the radical historical changes going on in European life: urbanization on a scale never seen before, explosive increase of population density, of the forces of production, of the volume of commercial transactions, of the means of transport and communications, reconfiguration of the work relations. The new form imposed on the human subjects submitted to the conditions of life in the mass age—the form of Mass Man—presupposed a previous form which would be superseded, and this was the initial form projected and dreamt of by the optimistic pioneers of the modern age: Man as an early modern ideal. What were the main features of this ideal?

Arguably the decisive keyword for introducing us into the essence of the early modern human ideal is *autonomy*. Early Modern Man claims the right to being himself the legitimate source or fundament of his own life and world. Hence, the supportive—and at the same time restrictive—orientations stemming from tradition and social conventions are refused, negated in favor of the undisputable sovereignty attributed to *reason*, *free will* and *experience* in determining one's choices, values and life projects. As a result, individuality (as opposed to the submission to collective traditional norms) becomes the highest value. And reflexivity is enthroned as the supreme guide in life. All these features are subsumed under the notion of autonomy, which etymologically means the property or capacity of one giving one's own laws.

The novelty in the early modern conception of autonomy (as distinct from the same notion as lived in antique philosophy) is that those laws are to be found exclusively inside oneself, inside one's *Self*. In the ancient form of mind, there was a *cosmo-logical* ethical and metaphysical significance of nature, so that the reflecting subject achieved his *autonomy* in rationally grasping the objective laws inscribed in the weft of the *cosmos*, within which he found his legitimate and ordered place, and in conforming his life to those objective cosmological/natural laws, as applied to his particular situation in the cosmic order. In the modern frame of mind, the notion of *cosmos* becomes obsolete, losing its former ethical and metaphysical relevance. Consequently, the human guiding laws (*nomoi*) can only be grounded and reflectively found inside one's *Self* or *subjectivity*, which is then the notion that summarizes the early modern definition of *Man*.

In modern philosophy, "*subjectivity*" in general designates "*self-consciousness*, thought of as that which is the most essential in the human being".[40] Yet subjectivity can be conceived of in two complementary ways: individually, meaning the interiority of the person, all that constitutes his/her individuality, and generically, meaning the pure self-consciousness (or reflexivity) present in every human being, fundament of every possible knowledge.[41] The former definition is usually referred to as the "empirical subject", whereas the latter is commonly known as the "transcendental subject". These two conceptions of subjectivity are *complementary*, which means that one should not simply oppose them as excluding one another. Dialectically, we could say that the universality of the transcendental subject shines in the singularity of the individual.

The transcendental subject does not express itself only in concrete individuals as empirical subjects; it is found first and foremost in the objective impersonal works and institutions of culture which express the particular *ethos* of a human community. The individual member of a society becomes an *ethical subject* (or *agent*) insofar as his/her empirical subjectivity is consciously and voluntarily informed by the general rules, ideals and values which define the particular ethical profile of his/her community. Beyond this level in which the historical and cultural particularity of any human society can be observed, one can reflectively establish a phenomenology of the *ethos* in general and after-

---

[40] E. Faye, entry "subjectivité", in A. Jacob & S. Auroux (dir.) *Encyclopédie Philosophique Universelle. Les Notions Philosophiques, Dictionnaire. Tome II.* Paris: P.U.F., 1990, p. 2477 (my translation). The philosophical approaches to "subjectivity" are extremely complex and diversified. Here I will make only a very meager and simplified *en passant* remark, as my purpose is only to make a bridge to the phenomenological description of "Mass Man".

[41] See ibid.

wards, through a transcendental reflection, disclose the transcendental level which constitutes the condition of possibility of *any* ethical life whatsoever.

As a rule, there is a coordination between the situation of the empirical subject and the cultural avatars of the transcendental subject, so that the individual finds the ways of his/her self-realization within the particular ethical parameters of the social human community to which he/she belongs (even when this self-realization requires *transgression* of given ethical limits, a possibility included in the phenomenology of the *ethos* under the concept of *ethical conflict*). The private, particular life is supported by the social sphere.

Now, precisely here we may find the essential articulation which enters in a state of crisis in modernity, giving rise to the predicament that accompanies the eventful history of the modern form of consciousness. For, under the concrete conditions of existence established in the wake of the Industrial Revolution, we recognize not anymore a *coordination* between the spheres of the transcendental I in its impersonal objective incarnations and the empirical individual with his/her subjective needs, but a radical *split*, so that the empirical I, surrounded and captured by the great impersonal systems of knowledge, economics and technology, is not able to find room in those systems for a *truly personal* self-realization. Therefore, the individual is confronted with a dramatic dilemma: either sacrificing his/her personhood in order to render possible the adaptation to the world as it is configured, or preserving it but paying the price of living in an artificial uprooted bubble in which self-realization may be enacted. The first option, which imposed itself historically, means bidding farewell to all the previous conceptions, developed throughout Western civilization, of what a true *human* existence was. The individuals are now irrevocably thrown into the status of *Mass Man*. In short, this means that the objective form of our industrial and post-industrial world leaves no room for the traditional idea of *Man*. It is *post-human* in its very logic.[42] Consequently, the classical and early modern notion of *Man* is rendered logically obsolete. "Man" as subjectivity, self-consciousness and reflexivity is substituted by a new form of being-in-the-world: the end of *Man* is tantamount to the birth of *Mass Man*. This means that the adjective "mass", as used here, should not be understood as designating a special class—the workers—but instead as referring to "a kind of man to be found today in all social classes, who consequently represents our age, in which he is the predominant, ruling power".[43] Mass Man corresponds to a form of consciousness in which the individual is utterly generic, and nothing but generic, having on principle no distinctive features which would differentiate it from all the others. The individual thus created is logically *absolutely identical* to everyone else: Mass Man is wholly and exclusively com-

---

[42] Objectively speaking, i.e., from the viewpoint of soul's *opus magnum*, it doesn't matter whether one is an enthusiastic functionary of the impersonal systems, or lives in an alternative community avoiding the constraints of modernity, or is the last remnant of an archaic people still not destroyed and/or assimilated by the course of Western modern civilization (for instance, some groups of the Yanomami, of northern Brazil). In all these cases—the happy acceptance of the new status, the hopeless heroic fight against it, or the innocent and blessed unconsciousness of it (which, however, must be *protected from it* in order to not being destroyed/transformed, as happened to many other non-European "archaic" people throughout history)—the supreme modern post-human rule dictates the conditions of life.

[43] José Ortega y Gasset. *The Revolt of the Masses*. New York: W.W. Norton & Company, 1932, p. 108.

prised by the sheer repetition of a generic type. Hence subjectivity and individuality become simply obsolete, and even tend to be annihilated. From this perspective, one can see that Mass Man is not a simple differentiation within the status of Man, but a true revolutionary change which throws away the variegated traces of humanism that were constitutive of the early modern ideal of Man.

We can make a brief outline of mass-mindedness and Mass Man's psychic condition through a few essential features.[44] Mass existence displays an amorphous kind of sociability, having as its principles the social *atomization* (the bonds between the individual and the group are systematically, programmatically wiped out) and the ensuing extreme *individualism* (collective interests are no more *truly* taken into account: all what one finds is a chaotic heap of individual interests). It could seem that mass-mindedness and individualism would exclude one another. But individualism not only did not prevent, but many times encouraged the self-abandonment into the mass. Why? Precisely because of the common ground underlying and uniting modern individualism and mass-mindedness: the complete *loss of roots*, of communitarian bondage, resulting in a deep seated and desperate sense of *superfluousness* and unbearable solitude. One of the chief characteristics of the Mass Man is his isolation and lack of what had previously been considered normal social relationships.

---

[44] In what follows I substantially rely on Hannah Arendt's reflections on this topic, as presented mainly in her important work *The Origins of Totalitarianism*. New York: Schocken Books, 2004.

Given that subjectivity is not a thing or a substance, but the dynamic synthesis of intersubjective relations,[45] how can one extinguish more efficiently the human subjectivity? By isolating it from other subjectivities, by rendering impossible the experience of mutual recognition, by destroying the bonds which make intersubjectivity possible in the first place, creating thus an aggregate of atomized so-called "individualities", mass men. This aggregate is only held together by the power of an impersonally fabricated system which encompasses all individual atoms in a whole and creates the surrogate to the lost sense of being at home, of having a world and a place in this world. These individual atoms are not anymore *subjects*: they are *objects* created by institutions which do not include or depend on subjectivity, but tend to subdue and to destroy it, even when not in an ostensible form. In the Mass Man status, the empirical individual is an objective thing. Moreover, the atomized individual position within the aggregating fabricated system shows that mass existence is fundamentally *abstract* (in the Hegelian sense).

The rise of the masses and the birth of Mass Man have an essential connection with scientificality. Technology is the grounding root from which mass society grows, and technology is essentially linked to scientific knowledge. Consequently, mass-mindedness and mass propaganda—a powerful means of molding collective consciousness—are

[45] The essential truth of subjectivity is not in solipsism, but in intersubjectivity. The human being only becomes a subject when in relation with other subjects. Subjectivation depends on the prior intersubjective field. Moreover, as subjectivity is not a fixed result, but an ongoing *dynamic* synthesis stemming from intersubjective relations, it only persists while the web of these relations is effective.

based on ideological *scientificality*, a feature of Western mind rooted in the primacy granted to scientific rationality in the modern constitution of consciousness. The techno-scientific mode of consciousness is structuring and exemplary to the mass-minded form of being-in-the-world. There is a strict correspondence between the specialization and growing fragmentation within the unlimited field of scientific knowledge and the social atomization of the individuals in the sociological sphere. Speaking from a classical humanist standpoint, Ortega y Gasset states that

> experimental science has progressed thanks in great part to the work of men astoundingly mediocre, and even less than mediocre. That is to say, modern science, the root and symbol of our actual civilization, finds a place for the intellectually commonplace man and allows him to work therein with success. The reason of this lies in what is at the same time the great advantage and the gravest peril of the new science, and of the civilization directed and represented by it, namely, mechanization. A fair amount of the things that have to be done in physics or in biology is mechanical work of the mind which can be done by anyone, or almost anyone. For the purpose of innumerable investigations it is possible to divide science into small sections, to enclose oneself in one of these, and to leave out of consideration all the rest. The solidity and exactitude of the methods allow of this temporary but quite real disarticulation of knowledge. The work is done under one of these methods as with a machine, and in order to obtain quite abundant results it is not even necessary to have rigorous notions of their meaning and foundations. In this way the majority of scientists help the general advance of science while shut up in the narrow cell of their laboratory, like the bee in the cell of its hive, or the turnspit in its wheel.[46]

[46] Ortega y Gasset, *The Revolt of the Masses*, pp. 110-111.

Hence, "the actual scientific man is the prototype of the mass-man".[47] And the ideological scientificality has a very precise function within the psychic condition of mass existence: it corresponds to the sore needs of homeless uprooted masses, insofar as it promises a reintegration "into eternal, all-dominating forces which by themselves would bear man, the swimmer on the waves of adversity, to the shores of safety".[48]

Uprootedness and *homelessness* are essential features of mass-mindedness. They engender a desire to escape from reality. This desire is fed by a deep rooted human need: the need of overcoming the chaotic and accidental conditions of life into a human fabricated pattern of relative consistency.[49] How this escape is accomplished? By channeling Mass Man's "longing for fiction", through an undisputed *privilege of imagination*, into an artificial paradise: a fabricated *fictitious* world. Masses are not convinced by facts, and not even by invented facts, but only by the consistency of a system which absorbs them.[50] This is one of

[47] Ortega y Gasset, *The Revolt of the Masses*, p. 109.
[48] Arendt, *The Origins of Totalitarianism*, p. 461.
[49] In the documentary *Matter of Heart*, as was mentioned on chapter 1, Marie-Louise von Franz deplores this tendency of escaping from reality, which she attributes to "young people". What she could not see was that it was a more universal tendency, rooted in mass existence. According to my interpretation, it is highly significant that she mentions this tendency in the context of Jung's final catastrophic vision of "the last fifty years of humankind".
[50] Consistency is the antidote for insecurity and uncertainty. Describing the "spiritual problem of modern man", Jung stated that "modern man has suffered an almost fatal shock, psychologically speaking, and as a result has fallen into profound uncertainty", (*CW* 10, § 155) and that "the upheaval of our world and the upheaval of our consciousness are one and the same." (*CW* 10, § 177) No wonder that his psychological project aimed at countering the overwhelming contemporary tendency

the "chief characteristics of modern masses": they "do not believe in anything visible, in the reality of their own experience; they do not trust their eyes and ears but only their imaginations, which may be caught by anything that is at once universal and consistent in itself".[51] This is the source of the "post-truth" mindset, with its proclivity to believe in adequately created "fake-news". The psychic gain of all this process is a restoration, on a different level, of what had been lost through massification: in a fabricated world of consistency, imagination properly manipulated gives to the uprooted masses a feeling of being at home, of being protected against shocks coming from real life and real experiences.

The trust in experience, one of the backbones of the modern mind, is abrogated in favor of *identification with the consistent fictitious system and total conformism of consciousness*. In fact, the very capacity for experience is numbed and rendered irrelevant in mass existence. Truly spontaneous experience is replaced by *programmed performance*. The more fanatic the adhesion of the individual to the fabricated system, the less can he or she be reached either by experience or by argument. The deliberate refusal of attending to the summons of reality results in the substitution of the living cognitive relation with reality by tightly programmed, standardized and codified forms of expression.

Along with the decline of the trust in experience, there happens also a subtle or veiled change in another

---

towards mass-mindedness (as becomes crystal clear in his essay "Present and Future" included in *CW* 10), and he presented *individuation* as the way to avoid this tendency.

[51] Arendt, *The Origins of Totalitarianism*, p. 462.

backbone of modern subjectivity: freedom. As Umberto Galimberti states: in the context of the mass society, "the actions of the individual are not read anymore as expression of his/her identity, but as possibilities calculated by the technical apparatus, which not only foresees them, but prescribes even the form of their execution. (...) the personal identity becomes sheer *functionality*".[52] Hence, the Mass Man is not anymore a man defined by the early modern sense of "self", becoming instead nothing but a *functionary of the system*. And as the functioning of the system obeys to fixed rules, freedom does not apply to the activity of its functionary.

The peculiar selflessness of the Mass Man can be grasped both in the yearning for anonymity and in its apparent opposite: the yearning for celebrity through visibility, as happens in the mediatic society, which reveals, nonetheless, that the sense of identity is exteriorized in the objective system of the media (according to the new proposition: "I am seen, therefore I am"). In both cases, the selflessness is evident, as well as the correspondent *suppression of true thinking*. Hannah Arendt summarized this feature of the condition of Mass Man by stating that he simply *cannot think* (and thinking is one of the essential activities that define the *human* life of the mind, according to the tradition to which Hannah Arendt affiliates herself).

The irrelevantification of the personal individuality in Mass Man condition gives rise to a typical feeling of *superfluousness*, which can be transformed in sheer contempt for the value of human life (as happens in State totalitarian-

---

[52] Umberto Galimberti. *Psiche e Techne. O Homem na Idade da Técnica.* São Paulo: Paulus, 2006, p. 19, my translation.

ism, this nearly perfect form of mass existence). Uprootedness is the preliminary condition for the feeling of superfluousness and the consequent devaluation of human life. And this psychic phenomenon is expressive of the objective *worthlessness* and ensuing *replaceability* of the individual in mass society.

The exemplary case of Mass Man directly examined by Hannah Arendt was the German Nazi leader Adolf Eichmann.[53] She observed in him the prominent features of vanity, exhibitionism, presumption, true thinking replaced by an ensemble of clichés programmed and implanted by the ideological atmosphere, a terrifying superficiality, an extraordinarily banal personality, wholly engulfed by the promptings of the system and thus ready to perform evil with banality, incapable of a true moral attitude and hence immunized against moral conflicts. In mass-mindedness, a human being is not considered as an end in itself, but as a means or instrument in view of the system. It is telling, in this respect, that Eichmann defended himself, justified his actions, by simply appealing to his position in the Nazi collective order: the ethical judgment was substituted by sheer conformism to rules prescribed by the system. Thus, in him we find the paradigmatic embodiment of the post-human condition of the individual as a functionary of the system, this being his new essential definition. In order to be transported to this new condition, the individual should be previously emptied out of all the former human essential features. From the destruction of "Man as reflecting subject" is born "Mass Man". In other words: mass-mindedness im-

[53] See Hannah Arendt. *Eichmann in Jerusalem. A Report on the Banality of Evil.* New York: Penguin Books, 1994.

plies a revolutionary transformation in the very nature of human being.

Another feature of mass-mindedness is *activism*, a feature that is preserved from the inner constitution of the early modern form of consciousness and transformed during the rise of mass society. Following Peter Sloterdijk's convincing remarks on the "irreflexive energies" at the base of the modern "ontology of the headstart",[54] we can say that the *primacy of the deed* is a structural feature in the modern form of consciousness. Activism defines the character of Goethe's Faust, this veritable symbol of modern man, and its foundational significance as modern consciousness' *arché* is emblematically expressed in Faust's famous translation of the first words of St. John's Gospel: "*Im Anfang war die Tat*" ("In the beginning was the Deed"). Activism, expressing the essentially modern "vocation to dishinibition", requires the throwing off of "the restrictive power of morality and convention".[55] Therefore, activism is consistent not only with the decline of reflexive thinking, but also with the widespread crisis of the effectiveness of moral values (the so called "ethical crisis of contemporary world").

The significant shift that activism receives in the transposition to the new mass form is that it migrates from the subjective sphere and effectively realizes itself in the objective form of the world, becoming thus a structural element of the world's great impersonal systems. The individuals (as well as the State and the companies) are much more captive victims of the whirlwind of economic and

---

[54] See Peter Sloterdijk. *In the World Interior of Capital*. Cambridge: Polity Press, 2013, pp. 66-76.
[55] Sloterdijk, *In the World Interior of Capital*, p. 74.

technological activism then its source. The Faustian *Streben* (a restless aspiration) becomes the omnipresent, impersonal and objective living spirit of our age. We could here remember Faust's bet with Mephistopheles: he is confident that a "poor devil" will not be able to provide him with anything that would satisfy his *absolute aspiration* (an aspiration to the Absolute, at bottom) so that he would want to stay in that moment forever. Consequently, without a real Absolute to match the Faustian aspiration, one is left with the infinite motion or "bad infinity" (Hegel) of a desire which, to apply Sartre's famous sentence on man, is a useless passion. In this way, we can see that contemporary activism is an effect of metaphysical nihilism.

As activism is essentially *movement*, its essential impetus creates *impermanence*. Conversely, impermanence is the condition of possibility for activism. This circularity between activism and impermanence is the secret of the *stability* of movement as the deep rule of modern life. No wonder that the anti-innovatory stance of classical metaphysics is incompatible with the modern form of consciousness: "within a metaphysics of the completed world (…) any innovation arouses suspicion of diabolical originality".[56] Hence the Mephistophelian shadow-side of the modern form of consciousness: unbridled destruction faithfully follows activity for the sake of itself. When this feature ceases to be only a particular dimension of certain individuals and/or enterprises and becomes universally and effectively realized in the world, we are faced with an easily recognizable aspect of its contemporary dynamism: the perpetual-motion mania, responsible for setting and keeping eve-

[56] Sloterdijk, *In the World Interior of Capital*, p. 74.

rything in motion. Psychically, this structural objective dimension finds correspondence in two outstanding characteristics of the mass-minded form of personality: its "extraordinary adaptability and absence of continuity",[57] which determines the *end of personal identity*.

Mass-mindedness follows a totalitarian logic, despite the fact that historical totalitarianism is only a particular expression of it. Concrete totalitarianism—as expressed in nazism, fascism, communism (or "real socialism")—is just an extreme and perfect exteriorization of the general logic of mass-mindedness. It crudely and explicitly strives for annihilating the individual personality without killing the victim, thus producing the perfect atomic social particle. If we only see through the grotesque and oppressive explicitness which particularizes totalitarianism, we find the general logic of mass-mindedness, which has other kinds of concrete expression, more subtle, more sophisticated, apparently more "soft", but much more pervasive and insidious.

Usually one takes expressions such as "totalitarianism of technology", or "totalitarianism of the market", as mere figures of speech, based on some superficial and regional similarities between the cultural-historical phenomena of "totalitarianism", "technology" and "market". But this relation should be taken very seriously, as disclosing a real common ground, namely, the same logical ground of mass-mindedness. Despite the differences in the manifestation of these distinct phenomena, the soul logic governing all of them is the same. When this logic succeeds in effectively informing the real world in such a way that "market", "cy-

[57] Arendt, *The Origins of Totalitarianism*, p. 408.

bernetics" and "advanced technology" merge unrestrictedly with individual and collective existence, we reach the fully accomplished technological mode of being-in-the-world, which is thus the latest version of mass-mindedness. I will now just highlight some of the essential features of mass-mindedness presented before as they are actualized in its current moment.[58]

The negation of the realness or givenness of the world achieves its highest form in the *virtual space* within which we all now live in medial modernity. The status of being fabricated and/or fictitious is blatantly evident in the contemporary techno-environment. The consistency of the technical environment can be accounted for by the extraordinary enthusiasm with which millions of people devote themselves to the plugged *cyberlife*. Indeed, the almost magical accomplishments of science and technology give support to the ideology of the technical salvation of humankind, strengthening in the masses the willingness to be reintegrated into "eternal, all-dominating forces which by themselves would bear man (…) to the shores of safety"—techno-scientific forces, of course.

On the other hand, the lack of concern for collective human interests and human welfare, a typical characteristic of the masses, which are not "driven by the famous instinct of self-preservation", having simply "drifted from mere concern with interest",[59] is exemplarily confirmed by the fact that the threat of planetary collapse, with the resulting

[58] For a brief indication of how, in contemporary phenomena, one can verify the end of the autonomous individual in our world, see Giegerich. *CEP V*, p. 375-369. (I am indebted to Greg Mogenson for having called my attention to this passage.)

[59] Arendt, *The Origins of Totalitarianism*, p. 458.

extinction of humanity, does not prevent mass society from continuing on the self-destructive course of the consumerist way of life. The contempt for any *human* interest reveals the post-human anti-utilitarian bias of mass-mindedness' logic.

Early modernity was to some extent conservative, insofar as it preserved many of the human values and ideals of the antique and medieval civilization: its notion of Man or subjectivity was not wholly other with regards to the classical and Christian definition of human being.[60] On the other hand, the latest phase of modern consciousness, in the moment of mediality, is quite different in that it entirely dispenses with all the previous human values constitutive of Western *ethos*: it is radically a post-human form of consciousness, and as such it disrupts the variegated line of Western humanism.

What happens now is a radical transformation in consciousness itself: it is changed into mere *awareness*. This can be confirmed in the primacy conceded to the here and now and in the correlative importance of the sensual impression and its emotionalized intensity, both informed by an *imaginative design* (which prescribes the form, meaning and value of the sensual impression and the corresponding emotions). This essential aspect of today's form of consciousness (as actualized in the Internet surfing, for instance) is what leads Wolfgang Giegerich to say that "in a way, it seems that today's consciousness has regressed to the very first status, that of 'sense certainty', of Hegel's *Phenomenology of Spirit*".[61] This regression is logically

[60] This can be easily confirmed in the first humanist moment of Feuerbach's thought, for instance.
[61] Giegerich. *CEP II.*, p. 328.

implied in mass-mindedness, but it has a distinctive feature, as we have seen: spontaneous experience is substituted by prefabricated performance. The primacy of sensual impression and emotions should not prevent us from seeing the underlying imaginative standardized "algorithm" which commands the performance in this regressive state of consciousness. Spontaneous sensual impression is virtualized, and this brings about a radical change in the very nature of experience.[62]

Reflexivity is congealed in a state of suspension and substituted by a standardized (even if very complex) data processing, as spirit becomes information and activism establishes itself as the perpetual-motion logic of the world. The frenetic movement is what renders reflexivity obsolete. The action of reflecting requires a halt and a turning back to an already finished event, or at least to a finished moment of an ongoing event. As such, reflection requires *memory*, and memory, as Augustine has taught us, is the way through which in the *present* we can experience—and reflect—the *past*. Past phenomena are *collected* and *immobilized* in memory (in the sense of being preserved from the actual dispersion in time, from sheer *annihilation*), and this is the *condition sine qua non* for their being reflected, thought: sheer nothingness subtracts itself from thinking. But the primacy of the "Now", imposed by the technological activism ruling the current mode of consciousness, in its specific form of "killing time", inevitably destroys memory. Through this active killing, time—the moving image of

---

[62] On this revolutionary impact of technology on sensation and experience as it can be verified in the phenomenon of television, see the comments of Wolfgang Giegerich in *CEP II*, pp. 302-305.

eternity, according to Plato—is interiorized as the *increasingly accelerated* perpetual-motion dynamism characteristic of the emptied form of temporality objectively informing consciousness today.[63] As a result, this consciousness deprived of the minimal stability of the past, of *memoria*, enraptured by the frenetic kind of movement generated by this form of killing time, simply cannot reflect, cannot think in the traditional sense of the word.

True reflexive thinking demands time—time for reception, for conception, for maturation, for making of a truth one's permanent possession, for becoming one with one's truth. The rule of accelerated movement, change, impermanence, hinders all these constitutive acts of thought. There is no more the required temporal conditions for truly *intelligere* (to understand, equivalent to *intus legere*, to read inwardly, to reach the interiority of a phenomenon),[64] but

---

[63] In archaic cultures the ordinary (and annihilating) flux of time is *recurrently* killed through rites, which actualize and make present the special time of the origins, the mythical (not natural) past, the *illud tempus*, a time which is not time. In other words: the immobilized eternity which thus triumphs over time. This is the metaphysical condition for *Meaning*. By contrast, in the "Now" instituted by the contemporary post-metaphysical "killing of time" one has a *mobile* surrogate of eternity, which is in fact an on principle increasingly accelerated movement striving helplessly and contradictorily to reach the absolute in movement itself. The nihilistic erasure of eternity enthrones time as the sole reference to consciousness. It is tantamount to the erasure of the Absolute.

[64] See St. Thomas Aquinas, *Summa Theologica*, II-II^{ae}, Q. 8, art. 1, respondeo. In the first moment of the modern psychological initiation of consciousness, "*initiation*" meant "one's being initiated through one's absolute-negatively interiorizing the phenomenon one is dealing with into itself and thus releasing it into its spirit and truth." (Giegerich, *WIS*, p. 321) This psychological consciousness now becomes logically obsolete, as there is no inner depth or inner infinity (no verticality) to be

only the increasingly faster and external stimulation by the flow of information. The objective restlessness and speed of the world find their perfect correspondence in the floating nature of consciousness when wholly immersed in the technological dynamisms. The remaining reflexivity is only a remnant from the superseded previous form of soul as subjectivity.

Therefore, true thinking ceases to be a collective regulative ideal and becomes a private option, objectively irrelevant. The new ideal is the expertise in data processing, reinforcing standardized forms of expression. Moreover, the triumph of the immediacy of image over the reflexivity of concept is a clear sign of the twilight of reason (with the exception of the instrumental and scientific modality of reason) and the consequent change in the form of conscious functioning.

Correspondingly, an unbelievable degree of banalization, frivolity and superficiality in consciousness is evident everywhere: TV, movies, newspapers, in the "personal" compulsive communications through any of the disposable means nowadays. Exhibitionism is *systematically* reinforced (meaning that it belongs to the logic of the system).

In the medial moment of mass-minded modernity, the obsolescence of the notion of truth and the hegemony of appearance through images render the latter the norm for personal identity (see Second Life, Facebook, etc.), whereas activism illuminates the fabrication of this same identity as a feature of today's society. The consequence is that the distinction between "true" and "false" self tends to become

---

disclosed in the web of horizontal phenomena in which we all live in the Age of Technique, also the age of the World Wide Web.

irrelevant. "Human nature" or "essence" was the referent for "true self"—so that one could define self-consciousness as the form of "human essence". But in the technological contemporary mode of being-in-the-world, which conjugates a) the transformation of nature into mere raw material to be disposed of by the technological activity, b) the obsolescence of the category of "essence", and c) the increasing (or almost complete) technical fabrication of the human environment (technique invading even the realm of human relations), the "true self" loses its grounding reference: from now on, *everything* is fabricated, including the self. Instead of "Become such as you are" (the maxim which ruled self-realization, or "individuation", since Ancient Greece), the driving maxim today is "Become what you want to be". This is the correlate of the hegemony of technology in today's world. The question is displaced from "Who am I?" to "Who do I want to be?" And the answer is to be found not anymore inside oneself, but in the varied and nevertheless calculated possibilities prescribed by the market.

When mass society assumes the form of the consumerist way of life, the consequence is that, "giving the false impression of replenishing the individuals with possible worlds, of multiple identities and choices always reversible, the culture of consumption spreads, in the propagation of those possibilities, that freedom which is seen, subsequently, as an abstention of the choice, typical in the world of conformism. As it is not associated to images of oppression, this form of lack of freedom is not perceived in the least, and the consequent deprivation that it entails is not followed even remotely by the sensation of being deprived of something".[65] Conformism, thus, imperceptibly extinguishes freedom and numbs consciousness. An at bottom "open conformism" is presented as the new form of freedom: the apparently free choices in determining one's "personalized" style of "costumerized" existence. This "personalization" tends in fact to create isolated individualistic bubbles (as is evident in the algorithmic functioning of the search programs in the Internet), and as such it is the new powerful way of producing the atomized individuality which is correlative of mass-mindedness.

Finally: needless to say, the accelerated movement and the perpetual-motion mania, which Hannah Arendt attributed to totalitarianism, are *a fortiori* extensible to the technological way of contemporary life. The above-mentioned sublation of activism into the syntax of the world of consumption and technological innovation is so obvious that it dispenses any further commentary.

The Riddle of Modern Consciousness: the Hidden Logical Source of Mass-mindedness

The rise of mass-mindedness was not just a historical accident in the course of Western civilization. As a matter of fact, the end of Man, in the sense here employed, is a logical event already implied in the very grounds of modern thought. There we can find the logical premise for the later actual historical rise of Mass Man—who, in all regards, is the surrogate of Man as defined in the classical Western notion of human being. This premise lies in the radical re-

---

[65] Galimberti, *Os Vícios Capitais e os Novos Vícios*, p. 77, my translation.

casting of the field of knowledge after the Middle Ages, and especially in its incidence in the ethical horizon, as it was established in Ancient Greek philosophy, particularly in Aristotle's *Nichomachean Ethics*. As is well known, Aristotle distinguished the spheres of *theoria* ("contemplation", as the disposition of human spirit aiming at pure knowledge, knowledge having as its exclusive goal knowledge itself, encompassing the theoretical sciences of metaphysics, physics and mathematics), *praxis* ("action", of a specifically human and humanizing kind, aimed at the perfection of the human agents themselves, both individually and as a community, and referring to the kind of knowledge oriented to *ta anthropina*, "things human", in the light of *arete*, "virtue" or "excellence", and encompassing the practical sciences of ethics and politics), and *poiesis* ("production", aimed at the perfection of an external work, encompassing all the technical knowledges and skills, in the broadest sense). This classical division of the sciences will suffer a veritable upheaval at the dawn of modern times.

The anthropological turn which inaugurates the modern mindset expresses itself as an inversion with regards to the former metaphysical foundation of knowledge. To understand this inversion, we must then first turn back to Ancient Greece in order to grasp the foundation which would be subverted in modern times. We can locate in Greek philosophy a fateful event, which was destined to have a long-lasting consequence: the historical triumph of a core metaphysical position of Plato over the one sustained by Protagoras. As we know from Plato himself (see *Theaetetus* 152a), Protagoras stated that "Man is the measure of all things". On the contrary, Plato explicitly rejected this anthropological foundation of knowledge and existence, and sustained a quite different position: "Now God ought to be to us the measure of all things, and not man, as men commonly say (Protagoras): the words are far more true of Him. And he who would be dear to God must, as far as is possible, be like Him and such as He is". (*Laws* IV, 716 c, trans. Benjamin Jowett). God is thus the exemplary measuring model, in relation to which all things are measured, including humankind, which finds its true realization in the likeness of this divine model. Plato's triumph over Protagoras heralds, on the realm of reason, the theological-metaphysical age of soul, sealing it with the stamp of transcendence.

The modern form of mind (which is made possible by previous discussions taking place in medieval scholastics) will be built upon an upheaval of the prevailing Platonic-Aristotelian metaphysical ground of thought. Subjectivity emerges as a new and valuable notion to express the essence of the nascent form of mind. It receives the primacy in the modern form of consciousness, and this form imposes itself as the organizing center of modern times in all its distinctive fields. Subjectivity is invested with the logical function of the Absolute, namely, being the metaphysical center around which all truths are established. This is a concise way of explaining the metaphysical meaning of the modern anthropo*centric* (or anthropo*logical*) turn, which precisely inaugurates the distinctively modern metaphysics of subjectivity: the modern notion of "Man", which is thus equivalent to the notion of "subjectivity", is the new logical or metaphysical center. Protagoras has resurrected.

In Descartes' famous "*cogito, ergo sum*", which represents the opening act of modern philosophy, we can grasp the radical move implied in the modern anthropological turn. In the Cartesian *cogito* we discern the inversion of the Platonic metaphysical axis, and the resurgence of a Protagorian-like position. True: still in line with the Platonic tradition, Descartes posits God as the fundament of the cogitating subject, after proving the existence of God as a (supposedly) rational requirement to fully account for the *cogito* (and the innate idea of "infinite"). But, on the other hand, Descartes's proof of the existence of God is logically dependent on the centrality of the cogitating subject, despite God being thought of as the fundament of the *cogito* (and as the guarantor of the reality of the physical world), for God *is a fundament required and posited by the subject*. Be that as it may, from Descartes to Hegel we find the rough line of evolution and fulfilment of the logical requirements constitutive of the truth of the modern form of consciousness. In short: from Plato until the modern times, the metaphysical center (or Absolute) was posited in "God;" the modern form of consciousness will gradually leave "God" aside and enthrone "Subjectivity" in its place (and Kant is the moment in this line of evolution where the anthropological requirement of the metaphysics of subjectivity comes home to itself, reaching the explicit and full consciousness of itself[66]).

However, this new foundation of metaphysics (this new form assumed by soul, or the new logical form of consciousness) has also an essentially different and decisive component: it is not sufficient to describe the logical status of modern consciousness by pointing to the metaphysical centrality assumed in it by subjectivity; one has to add to

[66] As becomes explicit with the reduction of the first three fundamental questions—What can I know? What ought I to do? What may I hope for?—to the fourth: What is Man?

the primacy of the transcendental subject, the primacy of a new and specific form of rationality. This form can be found in the new scientific spirit arising fully conscious of itself in Galileo: the new science on principle performs a *mathematization* of the real, and this is definitional to the modern meaning of science. This means that the ancient dialectics of the measuring and the measured, which opposed Plato to Protagoras, is now resumed in the modern New Science, but receiving an essential *mathematical slant of a purely geometrical-quantitative nature*, unheard of before.[67]

Equally decisive and innovative is the *instrumental* nature of this modern scientific knowledge: it is not merely *empirical*, but *experimental*, essentially allied to *technique*, and as such powerfully applied to the project announced in Descartes's *Discours de la Méthode*:

> For they [general notions from physics] made me see that it is possible to reach knowledges which would be very useful in life, and that in place of this speculative philosophy taught in schools, one can find a practical philosophy, by means of which, through knowing the power and the actions of fire, water, air, the stars, the heavens and all other bodies in our environment, as distinctly as we know the various crafts of our artisans, we could apply them,

[67] We should remember that in Plato's thought we find a kind of meta-mathematics of a distinctively *qualitative* nature, as is evident in his doctrine of *ideal numbers* (which should not be confused with the mathematical entities located at the lowest level of the intelligible realm). The absence of this qualitative dimension in the mathematical quantitative reduction informing the modern scientific spirit should make us take *cum grano salis* Alexandre Koyré's thesis about the supposedly Platonic metaphysical foundation of the New Science.

> like the artisans do, in all the appropriate ways, and thus make ourselves masters and possessors of Nature.[68]

This new "practical philosophy"—or scientific rationality—is thus explicitly *instrumental*: it does not aim at pure knowledge for its own sake, but seeks knowledge as a *means* for dominating and transforming nature. The theoretical dimension merges with the poietic. It is this essential alliance of science with technique (founding modern *technology*), under the aegis of the project of *domination of nature*, which renders obsolete the Aristotelian division of knowledge, and equally has the above-mentioned impact on ethical life. For, under the primacy now assumed by *techne*, the sphere of *praxis* will be swallowed, so to speak, by the sphere of *poiesis*. This has as an unavoidable consequence the transference of the ethical-practical normative knowledge of action (*praxis*, in the classical sense) to the realm of the technical knowledge of production (*poiesis*), entailing a redefinition of the notion of *praxis* itself: *praxis* "starts to be thought of under the basic category of the arithmetic equality that returns upon the agents, making them equal, and only differentiated by the simple number through which they are counted in the sequence of a numeric series".[69] Here is the deep logical premise which permits one to foresee the end of the classical notion of Man and the correspondent rise of Mass Man and mass society. From this logical root, one can see that the mass-minded form of consciousness is not "irrational" at all: it is extremely and

[68] R. Descartes. *Discurso do Método*. São Paulo: Martins Fontes, 2001, p. 69, my translation.
[69] H.C.L. Vaz. *Escritos de Filosofia II*. Ética e Cultura. São Paulo: Loyola, 1988, p. 111, my translation.

one-sidedly rational, informed as it is exclusively by the instrumental and mathematical kind of rationality. And this restricted form of rationality is on principle alien to the whole sphere of *ends*, meaning that it cannot provide them with a rational justification, it cannot ground them. The ends are simply given to it from outside, and then it finds the best means of actualizing them.

The suppression of the qualitative subjective aspects from the realm of true scientific knowledge and the correlative instauration of the "kingdom of quantity" define the new modern epistemological space. Only what on principle can be quantified and translated into mathematical language counts as a possible object for scientific knowledge. Consequently, also on principle modern science excludes the whole dimension of human intentions, values, virtues, ideals, brief: all what constituted the very specific and distinctive essence of "things human" (*ta anthropina*) in the classical notion of Man. We may say that the modern transcendental subject hosts a quantitative mathematician who handles only the instrumental kind of reason. This means that, in its very inception, the spirit of modernity brings within itself the self-contradictory tendency to destroy the classical idea of Man:

> Rabelais and all the humanist stream of Renaissance, prefacing the scientific flight and the scientism-based reduction of Western thought, already feared, long before Kant and the modern Times, this inescapable "laceration of consciousness", this "unhappy consciousness" dealt with by Hegel and whose misery results precisely from this deadly divorce, within man's reflection, between a science dedicated to a dehumanizing objectivity, and a consciousness in despair after being abandoned to dereliction, to a freedom incapable of settling the values and the

> will in a being whose perfection and existence were evident. The misery of modern consciousness is nothing but the acknowledgement of the annihilation of the subjective hopes, both individual and collective. Consciousness dies in the absence of a real land where it could grow, believe and embellish. And a science without consciousness is just this suicide of the singular being dissolved in objectivity, alienated from every difference and having no more a soil to root and realize its intimate hopes.[70]

To be sure, in its historical unfolding modern consciousness has gradually affirmed the humanist position implied in the anthropological turn and tributary of many features of the classical notion of Man. But the logical death blow on Man was from the outset included in its own structure, as a self-negating feature of the logical form of modern consciousness, pointing toward the post-human configuration. It is as if modern consciousness was logically pregnant with this new dehumanizing configuration. The occasion for the effective death of (classical and early modern) Man and the birth of its surrogate, Mass Man, presented itself in the beginnings of 19th century—all the external conditions for this radical event were finally achieved: the time was ripe, the historical labour would begin. From the Industrial Revolution onwards the instrumental rationality showed effectively its power in transforming the world. The impact on all cultural life was summarized precisely in the birth of mass society, with the correspondent mass-mindedness, and the simultaneous gradual decline of the humanist ideals.

Consequently, we have the paradox of modernity: built upon transcendental subjectivity, it corrodes its own

---

[70] Gilbert Durand. *L'âme tigrée*. Paris, Denoël, 1980, p. 13/14, my translation.

fundament and tends to the post-human constellation of the world as technical environment:

> The *riddle* of modernity is summarized in this fact: if, on the one hand, what characterizes modernity is the rise of a radically original subjectivity, on the other hand the growing primacy of techno-scientific rationality, inasmuch as it posits the horizon of *technical objectivity* as the all-encompassing continent of our being-in-the-world, leads to the forgetfulness of subjectivity itself and, consequently, to the decline of modernity itself. Therefore modernity, which on the one hand states the primacy of the subject, left aside the very subjectivity which defines modernity. As a consequence, post-modernity heralds itself in the form of nihilism.[71]

Nihilism is too broad a theme to be even superficially discussed here. Therefore, I will only recall its synthetic definition: the annihilation of any real Absolute (metaphysical nihilism), and the consequent impossibility of grounding any ethical order in a comprehensive notion of Being (ethical nihilism). After the closure of Hegel's astounding speculative effort, in which the Absolute was given its last monumental expression in thought, the realization of the "death of God" from Feuerbach to Nietzsche is correlative of the erosion of the category of the absolute. From now on, no more ground was possible. As Jung clearly saw, before the modern man "there yawns the void, and he turns away from it in horror" (*CW* 9i § 28).[72] Nihilism emerges both as

---

[71] C. M. Rocha de Oliveira. *Metafísica e Ética. A Filosofia da Pessoa em Lima Vaz como Resposta ao Niilismo Contemporâneo.* São Paulo: Loyola, 2013, p. 153, my translation.

[72] Also the "catastrophe in progress" in Jung's 1913 visions, which reduced civilization to rubble, and the "final catastrophe" in his last vision, which depicted the end of humankind, are imaginal expressions

the hidden plot and visible destination of the modern adventure.

However, nihilism is not just the final result of the historical unfolding of the modern form of consciousness, in its externalizations through the decisive moments of modern history. It is not due to accidental vicissitudes of historical experiences that the soul's logic prevalent in today's *opus magnum* is nihilistic. Nihilism is the deep seated truth of modern mind. It springs from its self-contradictory logical constitution. As such it gives the full meaning to those earlier alluded to "decisive moments of modern history".

The negation of the essential and foundational notion of Man, as a logical act (or moment) of modern soul's self-negation, bears upon the initial moment of its specific form of humanist consciousness. Western (Christian) humanism rests on the dignity attributed to the individual human person on account of its essential relation to God, the supreme value, a relation expressed in the theological idea of *imago dei*—the privilege of humankind being thought of as derived from its ontological constitution in the image and likeness of God. Philosophically, we can see the expression of this relation in the structural reference of Kant's moral agent to the ideas of freedom, immortality of the soul and existence of God (the postulates of practical reason). It can also be verified in the dialectical relation of human subjectivity to the Absolute according to Hegel. After Hegel, the absolute as such is dismissed in the logical setup underlying the industrial and post-industrial phase of modernity. Con-

---

of the nihilistic drive of modernity. The "yawning void" is fundamentally destructive.

sequently, the "death of God" is logically correlative of the "death (or end) of Man".[73] The former humanist dignity is simply emptied out, with the resulting consequence of the worthlessness of subjectivity, which is definitional in the new logical status of Mass Man. In the human agent we do not find anymore subjectivity as a privileged moment of the Absolute's self-manifestation and self-relation: the former subject is now nothing but a function in the impersonal systems of economics, knowledge and technique. From the new logical standpoint, the empirical subject is nothing but a functionary of the system—and as such replaceable, discardable, with no value of its own. Of course, there is always the possibility of the individual subject differentiating him/herself from the logic ruling the objective world, so as to become relatively emancipated from it. But this possibility does not affect the objective logical place reserved to humans in the wider sphere, regardless of whether one is privately engulfed and molded by the logic of mass mindedness or not.

The consummation of modernity (or its end) discloses a new level of consciousness, in which the absolute

[73] The Christian *kenosis* of God does not stop at the initial moment of incarnation, in the *birth* as a human being. Within this new status, God has to *die* as a human being, and to die *as a human being*, death here being the total annihilation of the ontological constitution of human *being*. In an informal talk with a Jesuit theologian about the meaning of the Apostles' Creed passage: "He descended to the dead", I asked him why there was practically nothing written or thought about it. He answered that this was the darkest spot in all the incarnation process, where effectively and absolutely God dies, and the theological intelligence sort of "trembled" in face of it. Maybe we could understand the annihilation of any trace of human dignity in the form of Mass Man as the "trembling" absolute historical fulfilling of the Christian *kenosis*, when consciousness reaches the bottom of "the house of the dead".

logical sublatedness of subjectivity (both divine and human) appears as constitutive of the fully nihilistic soul truth of the real.[74]

---

[74] Jung's final catastrophic vision of the last 50 years of humankind is a dramatic depiction of soul's abrogating the anti-nihilistic intention of his psychological project as informed by the 1913 catastrophic visions and dreams. The opposition to nihilism—Nietzsche had already taught us—is itself simply a form of confirming nihilism reactively. On the other hand, the "destruction of humankind" portrayed in Jung's vision corresponds to a *logical* catastrophe, already realized implicitly in the very constitution of the modern form of consciousness, as I have indicated, and effectively accomplished in the twilight of Man and the correlative rise of Mass Man brought about by the Industrial Revolution.

Chapter 3
The End of Man Manifested in Soul's *opus parvum*

The concrete actualization of the end of Man (as a logical feature of the modern form of consciousness in its post-human moment) is a soul process occurring at the level of soul's *opus magnum*. Now, it is commonly held that there is an *absolute* disengagement between the levels of *opus magnum* and *opus parvum*. Ordinarily, this thesis may be accepted without reservations, as the phenomena belonging to the *opus parvum* level in their entirety have only private and subjective *relevance*. Furthermore, the thesis does not imply that we could or should think the reality of the individuals as not included in the "big picture"—this would be absurd, as it would mean denying the historicity and worldliness of the empirical individual consciousness, which is entirely formed within and by a certain human mode of being-in-the-world, whose historicity is consensually admitted and whose logic is precisely the logic of the "big picture". The processes which occur at the level of *opus parvum*—the individual person's efforts in the sphere of soul-making, individuation, and meaning making—are culturally preconditioned. This means that they cannot fall out of the logic of the age, following thus the patterns established in *opus magnum*.

As I said, ordinarily the reference of the smaller private affairs to the broader sphere of culture is negligible on all accounts. For instance: the private experiences of marriage, childbirth, sickness, death, love, work and so on, in all their particular unlimited variations. Even if such all-too-human situations are necessarily lived within the particular configurations of the cultural horizon of the individuals, we should not waste our time in trying to establish the connection of this ordinary kind of material to soul's *opus magnum*, because *in the modern form of consciousness* they have strictly private subjective *meaning*.[75]

On the other hand, while it is true that soul "wants to unfold and display its full reality in the empirical world and real life",[76] it is also true that this refers not only to the great works and institutions of culture, but to the empirical consciousness of individuals as well, at least to some extent and in varied ways. A soul truth "wants" to be "embodied or incarnated as a personal reality in people",[77] it has "to be turned into the very syntax or logical form of consciousness itself".[78] To the degree that an individual consciousness may be said to be truly contemporary, it must be informed by the contemporary logic that defines the current status of soul at large. It has to be initiated "into the cultural truth of the age, so that in addition to [one's] entering [one's] personal adulthood [one] might also become a truly *modern* adult".[79] In the absence of an explicit, spectacular and ritually exteriorized initiation nowadays, "[w]hen the develop-

---

[75] Whereas in other cultural contexts some of these same human experiences could in some cases be given soul relevance and be lived according to their mythic or religious meaningful patterns, in the modern form of consciousness, defined by its emancipation from soul, this is not possible anymore: all the events belonging to *opus parvum* receive no soul dignity, being psychologically irrelevant with regards to the broader sphere of soul's *opus magnum*.

[76] Giegerich, *WIS*, p. 43.

[77] Giegerich, *CEP V*, p. 101.

[78] Giegerich, *CEP V*, p. 107.

[79] Giegerich, *CEP V*, p. 76.

ment happens to be 'normal', people simply seem to absorb osmotically the truth of the age".[80] "Osmotically" means unreflectedly, unconsciously, or at best semi-consciously. This psychological absorption happens due to the immersion of the all-too-human sphere in the soul of the real, to its irrevocable worldliness, and if this osmosis happens at all, it is because the borderline between the two levels is permeable, permitting the smaller human sphere to be informed by soul's broader objective logical status. This is what may be called a one-way "*communication*" between the two levels.

However, when consciousness is truly *initiated* into the truth of the age it makes this truth its own conscious and reflected norm, instead of being just informed by it through an unconscious "osmotic absorption". This is the ultimate goal not only of traditional rites of initiation, but also of modern psychological work or soul-making, in whichever form it takes (art, philosophical thought, depth psychology etc.) The unconscious "osmotic absorption" is not the whole truth of the initiatory process in and into the modern form of consciousness. It lacks the self-conscious quality of the final result of the fully actualized initiation. The deepest purpose of true initiation is to make conscious the pervasive status in which consciousness is already unconsciously immersed and lives in, so that the truth of the age comes home to itself in individual consciousness, as its self-conscious syntactical pattern, as the *allowed* truth of one's life. We must remember that "[w]hat has factually happened requires, on top of its already being the case, to be explicitly

---

[80] Giegerich, *CEP V*, p. 76 note 9.

allowed to be the case and thus to become *true*. It has to be released into its being true. (...) Through a specific logical act of our own we have to own up to what our real situation is in order to make it true and in this way appropriate the factual situation as our own property, to make it psychologically our own. Psychologically, we have to still get to where we in fact already are".[81]

At this juncture, we should not ignore that a further problem arises here. Considering that any initiation whatsoever has the same syntactical structure (the move into the psychic other), "no matter in what cultural age under what circumstances, with what utensils and into which particular guise it takes place",[82] how could we possibly think an initiation into soul's truth of the age *in the modern form of consciousness*, once we admit that what characterizes this form is *emancipation from soul*? At first sight, it would seem impossible, as initiation is the opposite of emancipation, and thus would imply the abrogation of emancipation. Hence initiation, in the modern stance of consciousness, would be an exclusively private subjective process, ruled by the common syntax of any such transformation process, with the peculiarity of being simply and absolutely disengaged from the truth of the real, once modern consciousness is by definition emancipated from soul. Consequently there

[81] Giegerich, *CEP V*, p. 34. This is homologous to what, on a different (essentialist) historical context of soul, Greek poet Pindar expressed in his famous maxim "γένοι' οἷος ἐσσὶ μαθών" ("Become such as you are, having learned what that is", usually abbreviated as "Become what you are"), a maxim which, since Ancient Greece, has been indelibly inscribed within the ethical horizons of Western civilization.

[82] Wolfgang Giegerich, personal communication, 20 February 2014.

would be no full initiation into the soul truth of the age: only unconscious "osmotic absorption".

However, initiation into the truth of the age *does happen* in the modern form of consciousness. One does not only become a modern *adult*, but also a *modern* adult, and not only unconsciously. Accordingly, there are occasions in which we can clearly see an *opus parvum* event displaying the logic of the *opus magnum* process and explicitly manifesting the truth of the age in its semantic content. This was the case, for instance, with Jung's catastrophic visions and dreams in 1913/1914. That raw psychic material was an individual subjective phenomenon which clearly conveyed an impersonal, non-subjective *meaning*, wholly consistent with and expressive of the objective soul truth informing the historical situation at that time.

Another example may be helpful here to ground my claim concerning this problematic point. In his essay "Psychology as Anti-Philosophy: C.G. Jung",[83] Wolfgang Giegerich analyzes Jung's thought experience of the shitting God destroying the cathedral of Basel (a psychic event which could perfectly have happened as a dream as well). He sees in that event of thought a (failed) initiation into a truth of the age (namely, the ruin of the concept of God), so that Jung's "personal development was (implicitly) loaded with the problem of the *krisis* of two historical ages".[84] This is sufficient to prove that initiation into the truth of the age *can* happen in modern consciousness, and through an *opus parvum* event, "as a private spontaneous inner experi-

[83] In *CEP V*, p. 21-65.
[84] Giegerich, *CEP V*, p. 31.

ence",[85] by means of which the individual reaches simultaneously a logically *adult* and *modern* position of consciousness. Additionally, it confirms that the alluded disengagement between *opus parvum* and *opus magnum* is not absolute, and the one-way communication between the two levels can be verified and reflected, beyond the mere "osmotic absorption". In the case of Jung's inner experience, this communication is grounded in the thought-image of the "shitting God", which means the very destruction of the notion of "God", a soul truth of modernity.

Even if such cases are relatively rare, being rather the exception then the rule, they are sufficient to force us to relativize the *absoluteness* of the disengagement between *opus magnum* and *opus parvum* in order to account for such exceptions, but only *with regards to their meaning and logic, and not their relevance.* Jung's catastrophic psychic material, for instance, as any other *opus parvum* event, did not have relevance *in itself.* It was only an overwhelming and extraordinary psychic occurrence falling on a gifted individual. The (relative) relevance should be attributed to what this gifted individual, pressed by the promptings of soul, made of his private experience of the objective psyche: Analytical Psychology as a legitimate expression of the 20th century culture. But, on the other hand, the psychological depth of that psychic material revealed an *objective meaning* which was in direct correspondence with the logic prevalent in soul's *opus magnum.* That material can be said to have the same nature of an artistic vision (*Anschauung*), and as such it is not a product of Jung's ego concerns, relative only to his private affairs, but a thought produced by and in

---

[85] Giegerich, *CEP V*, p. 76.

him as *totus homo*. Consequently, the consciousness in the individual Carl Gustav Jung was moved *through* that experience, assimilating itself to its objective logic, positioning itself in relation to this logic, and additionally Jung succeeded in giving it an objectively relevant expression in his work.

As I see it, this exceptionally clear form of communication between the two levels of soul activity is one way that soul itself may take to *initiate* empirical consciousness into soul's current truth. The consequences of this initiation (whether there will be a transposition to the broader sphere of culture or just a private subjective transformation of consciousness) depend on factors and variables other than the psychic material itself.

As in modernity initiations are "no longer cultural institutions", they have to happen "as a private spontaneous inner experience". Now, I submit that this kind of initiation process does not have to be manifested only through extraordinary and bombastic psychic events such as Jung's visions, or his personally dramatic awakened thought experience of the shitting God, but also in some smaller material, in a more discreet and humble way. If this is so, then occasionally we may be able to observe the initiation of consciousness into the broader and deeper fundaments of modern culture manifested in the personal level, including in dreams. In this case, the subjective psychic material will have to have the same logical form of the objective psychological truth of the soul of the real. This coincidence *per se* allows for the objective truth of the age to graft itself in the subjective sphere, and this probably would be how the alluded "osmotic absorption" happens. But additionally, this logical coincidence also would have to be verified in its semantic expression (or refraction) in the subjective material, so that a self-conscious status of the truth of the age could be reached in the *opus parvum* level.[86] As an illustration of this possibility, I will now present and discuss an ordinary and wholly personal dream which—I submit—exhibits this kind of convergence of *opus parvum* and *opus magnum*, having an *objective meaning* and being thus a small piece of the potential initiation of the dreamer's consciousness in soul's objective logical status. This initiatory potentiality can be seen provided we adequately interiorize the dream image into itself, working it in the light of the basic assumptions of psychology as a discipline of interiority.

After an exchange of ideas about the symbolism of extraterrestrial beings (or aliens) as images of the Self, in the classical Jungian sense, a 39 years-old woman had the following dream: *the dreamer saw herself in a place with her working colleagues. There was a long queue, and the people were going to be transformed into aliens (E.Ts.), willingly. This was accomplished by each person connecting her/himself through wires to machines. And then they were transformed into compacted bricks of garbage. Seeing*

[86] Referring to the historical shift from communal, public knowing and truth to felt experience, Wolfgang Giegerich states: "This fundamental shift in the history of the soul that came about with its entrance into modernity (around 1800) had only 'implicitly', in the objective logic or syntax of modernity, become a reality. It also needed to become 'explicit' and semantic. What had become the logical truth of the individual also needed to be taken over by the *empirical* personality of the individual and established in it as a positively existing self-definition and way of experiencing itself." (*CEP V*, p. 264) This applies to the situation here discussed.

that, the dreamer was terrified, but people were calm, placid: that was what they wanted.

The important day residue included in the production of this dream has to be taken into account in its interpretation: an exchange of ideas, in which the image of the *alien* was envisaged as a "*symbol of the Self*", in old Jungian parlance, preceded the dream. In order to interiorize the dream image into itself, we have to approach it in the light of this connection, i.e., granting that the association alien-self belongs to the dream image, to its semantic content. If the dream action was "people connecting themselves through wires to machines in order to become aliens", and if that means "becoming self", then the self should be located both semantically (as a content of the dream text) and syntactically (as corresponding to its underlying logic) in the final result of the transformation presented in the *lysis* of the dream: in the "compacted bricks of garbage".

This alien-self is the result of a productive activity, which in the dream is performed by "machines". What kind of activity do the dream machines execute? One could be led to think that it is just a realistic, literal and non-problematic "compacting" activity, as happens in empirical trash processing. However, this is not what is going on in the dream, because in this case the "*garbage*" would remain unexplained, insofar as one should have "compacted bricks of *human flesh*" instead of "*garbage*". Therefore, there is a mysterious non-naturalistic process depicted in the dream, which is precisely the *transformation* of human beings into garbage.

This transformation happens through people's "*connecting* themselves to machines"—and, *nota bene*, the dream text does not say that they were "*compacting* machines". We should not break our rule of "not letting anything that does not belong come in" by assuming any kind of specific compacting machine as the cause of the compacting activity. This is not mentioned in the dream text, it "does not belong". Moreover, a real compacting machine does not work like that, it does not need to have the objects to be compacted connected to it through wires. No. The image is precise, self-sufficient and wholly symbolic. What happens here does not come from an empirical naturalistic referent: we are faced with a true *soul* process. Hence the connection and the compaction must be understood as what they truly express: a logical act of soul.

The transformation is a psychological deepening from ego as common human form to self as compacted brick of garbage. We must observe that the resulting subjective element itself is wholly affected, circumscribed and determined by the transformation, inasmuch as the garbage is *produced* by the compacting-transforming activity ensued by the connection to the machines, receiving its formal configuration from this symbolic "technological" process. The form of "*brick*" and the status of "*garbage*" are imposed by soul in the transformation process.

The transformation of the human form into some other ("alien") one is a common syntactical feature of the initiatory processes in general. In the context of shamanistic cultures, for example, the individual submitted to initiation usually is transformed into an animal—an eagle, or a bear, for instance. But in our dream we have a different situation. If the dream image was of people being transformed into *robots*, or *cyborgs*, the initiation would be strictly analogous to being transformed into an animal in the context of shamanistic cultures, as these forms of the psychic other are representative of the higher values and goals of the respective cultures (integration into the spiritualized nature, integration into the technologically conformed world), and the received non-human form would accordingly grant a higher value to the individual, raising him/her to the sphere of the soul fundaments of the community. But the representation of the psychic other as *garbage* implies a radical *devaluation* brought about by the transformation process. In order to understand this particular situation, we must first examine what are the essential aspects contained in the notion of "garbage", so that we can see the specific nature and moment of the initiation going on.

In the first place, garbage is defined by its *worthlessness*. It has no value, and hence it is meant to be *discarded*, thrown away, thrust aside, as it is also *useless*. Uselessness is an aspect of its worthlessness, and as such is attributed to garbage and constitutive of its concept. Uselessness, on its part, negatively refers to something else, to a context which defines what is valuable and useful, and what is not. In relation to this context, that which is considered as garbage is worthless, useless, unassimilated. In other words: garbage is essentially a form of *negative relatedness*.

We should note that in our dream the production of self as compacted bricks of garbage is the intended goal of the soul process. It is not accidental, and it is a complete transformation. In accordance with the internal psychic otherness which constitutes the *terminus ad quem* of the movement of transformation in any initiation, the relativity of self-garbage refers in the first place to the initial ego position (the form of people to be transformed). The self is garbage *to* the dream-I (meaning not only that she sees it as garbage, but mainly that it is offered to her as garbage). Usefulness, in the broader sense, is an essential criterion belonging to the pragmatic ego world. Consequently, the self in the dream as the ego's psychic other is worthless, useless and is meant to be discarded, thrown out. In its uselessness, "garbage" may thus be read as the semanticized expression of the absolute negativity of the self.

Therefore, we have here the depiction of the psychological difference,[87] and of the avertedness between soul and ego. Strictly speaking, the initiation in the dream is a personal initiation into the soul side of the psychological difference, and at a first glance can be satisfactorily understood within the limits of *opus parvum*. That which is presented to and refused by the dream-I is a change of the logical constitution of the I (from ego to self), performed through a kind of alchemical *putrefactio*.[88] Given the range of essential meanings implied in the notion of "garbage", it is warranted to state that the initiation offered in this dream

[87] The key concept proposed by Giegerich: the difference between the notions of "soul" and "man". As soon as the elaboration of the *Red Book* Jung had already formulated what is implied in the notion of the psychological difference: "From this we learn how the spirit of the depths considers the soul: he sees her as a living and self-existing being, and with this he contradicts the spirit of this time for whom the soul is a thing dependent on man" (Jung, *The Red Book*, p. 232). Consequently, "man" is not the ontic substrate of "soul".

[88] I am indebted to Wolfgang Giegerich for having called my attention to the alchemical analogy to this dream's transformation. He also recalled the designation of the alchemical stone as *lapis in via ejectus, vilis and exilis*, which provides a very good amplificatory context for the self as "compacted brick of garbage".

is an initiation into *the self as worthless, useless, in the status of discardedness*.

We know that the self as the internal other of the ego is "not-I", and "despite its otherness is nevertheless also I (me) (…) [and] is thus not self-identical and self-enclosed like an entity"[89]. In our dream the logical truth (the up to that point "undiscovered self") of the initial ego position is disclosed and expressed as "garbage". The transformation in the dream is performed on a *multitude of people* queued in line, which shows that it is a collective process, it involves a collective or common form of ego consciousness being transformed into *self*-consciousness (here meaning: consciousness as self-garbage). As the dream-I does not get in the queue, she does not permit herself to be raised (and dialectically lowered) to this self-consciousness. By resisting this transformation, she protects her highly valued ego position from being submitted to the syntactical putrefaction, dissolution. She rejects the thought of the logical worthlessness and discardedness of the self *as a personally valid truth, as the logical form in which she exists*. She excludes herself from this truth, denying it. But precisely because of this rejection, she remains tightly chained to what she rejects. She is defined by the rejection, *as* a rejecting subject. The dream-I only *recognizes* the truth, but does not let herself be submitted to it: she stays in *opposition* to it, *outside* it, not allowing to be affected by it in her subjective constitution. She does not "allow truth to be the case and thus to become true". Truth is seen only as an alien external reality, from a subject-object position. As such, the dream-I

[89] Giegerich, *WIS*, p. 298.

adheres to the *untruth* of her conscious position, and rejects the full consequences of the real dream-thought: there is no going under of the dream-I.

The self in the dream is presented as a very familiar and ordinary worthless element (garbage), and not in some semantic form which would stress its otherness (for instance: a monstrous imaginary extraterrestrial form of life). However, the compacted *brick* of garbage as a version of the alchemical *stone* is rejected not only because of its outward banal aspect (which leads the ordinary *vulgi* consciousness to despise it as nothing but an ordinary element of banal reality, and which clashes against the dream-I's position). Soul itself presents the self as worthless and discardable, as something ("garbage") whose essence or notion is to be actively rejected and discarded. Consequently, its rejection by the dream-I is not an ego mistake, but a reaction intended by soul itself.[90] It is indicative of the unallowed effective realization of the truth *in* the dream-I, happening though in the dialectical moment of first negation. The possibility of confrontation with this soul truth is reserved to the dream-I, who reacted and negated it. Without this reaction, there would be no truly self-conscious syntactical move. However, she will only logically "die" if she unconditionally submits herself to that truth, fully realizing it in herself. Furthermore, this would be a condition of pos-

[90] "We know from dreams that the degree of extremeness of an image simply reflects the degree of the dream I's resistance or lack of understanding. Through its disgusting, unpalatable character the image indicates within itself that this initiation *came* as one to be rejected." (Giegerich, *CEP V*, p. 86)

sibility to a further emancipation and differentiation of consciousness from that level of truth.

We could legitimately stop at this point the interpretation of this dream. However, given the previously alluded possibility that modern initiation, happening "as a private spontaneous inner experience", can have a particular broader reach so as to be simultaneously an initiation into a soul truth of the age, we can go a step further and see whether and how the thought expressed in the image of the self as "compacted brick of garbage" could allow us to think this particular personal initiation as being in effective communication with the soul fundaments of our world. Has the putrefaction depicted in our dream a *discernible objective real depth*, or is it only one moment, the first immediacy of a private potential initiation without any reference to the soul truth of the age?

Wolfgang Giegerich has called our attention to the fact that

> what is (consciously or unconsciously) in individual consciousness must before have been in a cultural institution or work (…) Consciousness (…) "de-pends" on or from the cultural products as its "extraterrestrial satellites" shot up into an orbit around the human "Earth". (…) Everything new comes from outside ("above") into consciousness. It first hovers "in the sky", as it were, and is marveled at and revered as something higher (*often, however, only after initially having been experienced as something threatening by consciousness, which therefore violently rejected it as a scandalous attack upon the culture's established familiar truth.*) And only slowly can it come down into people's consciousness as their inner possession (or part of the make-up of their personality), either through a "leap after the throw", i.e., a long process of integration of what had been "thrown" far ahead and up into

> the future, or through a gradual accustoming and sedimentation process that results in the new forms and ideas ending up as sunken cultural assets in people's inner.[91]

We can read one essential aspect of the dialectical dynamism of the historical self-transformation of soul in Western civilization from this perspective. As is well-known, and as I mentioned before, Western humanism is informed by the biblical and Christian theological notion of Man as *imago Dei*, and this particular historical notion endows human being with an extraordinary value and relevance, raising it above all other creatures. This value is strengthened by the Christian dogma of incarnation: God's *kenosis* deprives "God" of its sublime transcendent value, and at the same time it invests "Man" (the human condition, *sarx*) with an unheard of privilege. At the dawn of the modern times, the anthropological turn will provide a renewed version of this privilege. But in the logical shift implied in the Industrial Revolution, what formerly was a cultural truth and had been sedimented as sunken cultural assets in people's inner throughout history (specifically the high value attributed both to God and the subjective human interiority),[92] constituting the individual consciousness, is submitted

[91] Giegerich, *WIS*, p. 183 (italics mine).

[92] An example of this high value is in Augustine's so-called "metaphysics of interiority", a forerunner of modern metaphysics of subjectivity. Let us recall the famous passage of his *De Vera Religione*: "*Noli foras ire, in teipsum redi; in interiore homine habitat Veritas*" ("Do not go out of thyself, return to thyself; it is in Man's interiority that Truth resides"). Whereas in Augustine Truth (*Veritas*) constitutes human reason but is ultimately *transcendent* to it, in the modern metaphysics of subjectivity Truth is wholly coincident with immanence. In the modern

to putrefaction, is destroyed by soul itself (remember Jung's thought experience of the shitting God, as well as his final vision of the extinction of humanity), and a new logical profile is established on the level of soul's *opus magnum*, which could be expressed as the "death of God" and the correspondent "end of Man".[93] This new logical post-human configuration, which corresponds to the objective truth of our age (even as it refers to its realization in "people's consciousness as their inner possession"), is still in the slow process of integration and/or sedimentation, as very often it is still "experienced as something threatening by consciousness" and rejected as "a scandalous attack upon the culture's established familiar truth" in those cultural loci which are still influenced by the logically obsolete truth of the self as the highest human value. (All the vehement defense of "human rights" in our times is a cultural reaction *against* the empirical distorted consequences of the logical obsolescence of subjectivity, of the historical putrefaction of "Man".)

This highly valued status of human essence is in blatant and shocking contrast with our dream's depiction of the self as "garbage".[94] "Self", as an explicit topic for the

form of consciousness, Truth does not only dwell (*habitat*) in subjectivity: it *is* subjectivity.

[93] Jung's conception of the "true self as the God image inside oneself" leads to the logical consequence that the value of the individual (and of individuation as opposed to *massification*) only subsists in the *personal* relation to *God* (see his essay "Present and Future", in CW 10). What happens with this value (and with Jung's notion of individuation) after the ruin of the concept of "God"? It is also ruined. In other words: it becomes logically obsolete.

[94] Here it is worth mentioning the divergence between Catholic and Protestant understanding of the consequences of the "original sin". To Luther, sin has *erased* all value from human being (the *imago Dei* was

dream-I ("transformation into alien-self" is a semantic content of the dream), is implicitly seen from her initial perspective as something valuable—otherwise, why should the dream-I be shocked by the thought of the *worthlessness* of self and reject it? The ego position, in the present case (as in Jung's experience of the shitting God), has an underlying implicit correspondence to formerly established cultural truths, and it clashes against the new cultural (modern) truth which comes to supersede them. To be sure, we don't find explicitly "Man" in the dream. However, we do find "*self*" (as associated to "*aliens*", in "people wanting to become *aliens*"). Moreover, we find "self" *syntactically* in the dream (as the psychic other in the transformation process), and "self" by definition is precisely *not* the private individual, the narrow egoic subjectivity, designating instead the *historical locus* at which private individuals find themselves. The objective soul is always embodied, and receives its specific, particular form from the real time and place in which it manifests itself. And "self" reflects the condition of the objective soul at a given historical locus: soul as subjectivity (or self) corresponds to the early modern definition of "Man".

---

corrupted), whereas to the Catholic understanding sin only *obfuscated* the essential relation of human being to God, throwing a shadow (*umbra*) on it. In the Protestant stance, all value of human being was lost through sin; in the Catholic stance, it was essentially preserved. But according to the logic of both cases, if "God" is disinvested of the psychological value, "human being" is helplessly deprived of any possibility of having its value rescued. Therefore, from a theological standpoint the putrefaction of "Man" brought about by the logical obsolescence of "God" is identical to the absolutization of the consequence of original sin.

Therefore, in our small dream we can discern an objective correspondence with the ruin of the modern humanist concept of Man (the "end of Man"). This problem belongs to the cultural context of the dreaming consciousness, affecting the historical locus in which the dream takes place, inasmuch as the Christian values have been deeply sunken in Western consciousness (no matter whether the empirical individual is a believer or an atheist). The putrefaction in the dream and its rejection by the dream-I have to be understood in the dreaming consciousness' *Sitz im Leben*, with all the historical undertones that are implied in today's Western reality: the devaluation of self as worthless and discardable is in frontal opposition to the Christian and early modern sources of Western consciousness; therefore the sedimented subjective asset of Western humanism, in the form of the dream-I's initial implicit high valuation of self (at least of "*her*self"), is completely negated in the image of self as garbage. This conflict is implicitly hinted at in the dream, if we seriously take into account the postulates of psychology as a discipline of interiority concerning the historicity of consciousness and the immersion of the human sphere in the soul of the real.

Putrefaction, which in the dream involves the conscious position of the dream-I, is an all-too-common moment in the initiatory process in its alchemical version, and there is no inherent need to see it as necessarily connected to an aspect of the soul of the real. Subjectively speaking, the dream's initiation discloses the immunity of the dream-I *against* the truth that is already informing her position. But through the semantic singularity of the expression of the self as "compacted brick of garbage" we can discern a kind of intersection of a moment of the universal syntax of initiation (putrefaction, resulting in a devalued form of self) with a feature of the specific logic of modernity (the logical obsolescence of subjectivity and of individuation, with the consequent substitution by mass-mindedness). Consequently, the dream-I's resistance is directed against a truth that coincides with an objective aspect of the logic of the real, so that this dream must be interpreted as a moment of an all-too-common initiation, but at the same time as an initiation into an essential logical aspect of the modern soul of the real. It has an objective *meaning*. The *putrefactio* in the dream reveals the real immersion of the subjective sphere in the truth of modern age: it is a *modern* putrefaction. The initiation into the obsolescence, sublatedness, sunkenness of the self *is* an initiation into the objective logical status of human condition in the contemporary world. What was only an unconscious "osmotic absorption" of the truth of the age, or simply an idea that did not essentially touch the dreamer herself, is consciously reflected in the dream and establishes a conflict with the initial position of the dream-I by summoning her.[95]

---

[95] This conclusion could be charged of being nothing but an arbitrary result of an external reflection, not coming from the interiorization of the dream image into itself. I am not convinced that this is the case. It seems to me as being perfectly in tune with the sense of the initiation portrayed in the dream, and rooted in its own elements. It does not distort or inflate the dream, but only finds its deeper embedment in the real. As this further move (from the strictly private level of the dream to its being explicitly informed by the soul of the real) is liable to raise objections, let me stress once more that it is accomplished in strict observance of two basic postulates admitted in psychology as a discipline of interiority. If we think under the assumption that 1) "consciousness is, as it were, 'surrounded' by [the truth and soul of the real] on all sides as well as permeated and governed by it in all its acts", so that "all hu-

Considering that there is a gap or delay between the initial state of personal consciousness and the objective soul truth of the real, so that the initial relation of the former with the latter is that of an unconscious "osmotic absorption", and if psychologically "we have to still get to where we in fact already are", if the implicit logical truth of the individual also needs "to be taken over by the *empirical* personality of the individual and established in it as a positively existing self-definition and way of experiencing itself", then with regards to the logical status of human subjectivity in the broader sphere a *modern* individual subject may have to be initiated into its logical obsolescence, worthlessness, uselessness and discardedness, *provided the particular configuration of consciousness in him/her is still fed by a (logically obsolete) humanist pattern.* Now, the transformation displayed in the dream represents an initiation of the dream-I exactly into the worthlessness, uselessness and discardedness of self as "compacted brick of garbage". But this is precisely the logical status of self as subjectivity in the soul of the real today: it has no function or meaning in the broader objective soul context. This means that in the dream one finds a perfect correspondence with the ruin of the *modern* concept of self (which, being equivalent to subjectivity, was not only highly valued in the early modern form of consciousness, but also its logical center). This ruin may be understood as the truth of the subject as a "particle in the mass", the truth of the objective logical ob-

---

man world experience takes place within the horizon of this truth" (Giegerich, *WIS*, p. 197-198), and that 2) initiation means the coming home of this truth—which is a *cultural truth*—to the personal consciousness, then we are entitled to indicate if and how an initiatory dream may be *explicitly* related to the truth of the age.

solescence of subjectivity and its substitution by the form of Mass Man.

One aspect of the self as compacted brick of garbage deserves closer attention: its *discardedness*. This is a decisive detail of the dream image: the self, in its worthlessness and uselessness (it has no *use* in the pragmatic stance of the practical I), is produced *to be discarded.* The rejection is not only in the dream-I's refusal of the new form produced by the transformation: it is inscribed in the very form produced, as its own essence. The discardedness of the self is correlative of its fundamental *alienation* in relation to the ego world, of its being not-I. Thus it represents the inner relation of the two *relata* (I and not-I) constitutive of the psychological difference *within the level of soul's opus parvum*. On the other hand, insofar as self is *also* equivalent to soul as subject *as a whole* (and thus the dialectical unity of I and internal not-I comprising the entirety of the psychological difference), we can securely state that the worthlessness of self-as-garbage affects and qualifies the whole subjective sphere, the whole level of *opus parvum* as self-depicted in our dream. And as "garbage" implies the reference to a context which produces it and from which it is discarded, the discardedness of the self in our dream has a further amplitude: ultimately, it points to the alienation between the whole subjective sphere and the sphere of soul's *opus magnum*. In other words: self as "compacted brick of garbage" is the truth of the human sphere (at least a moment of this truth), which is thus worthless, useless and discardable in its entirety *in relation to the broader objective sphere.*

We know that individuation has become logically obsolete, and that "it occurs only *as* disconnected, disengaged from what psychologically is really going on in our age".[96] Our small dream is precisely an imaginal depiction of this logical status of individuation. The disconnection and disengagement of the subjective sphere from soul's *opus magnum* is equivalent to the discardedness of the self. As the *telos* of individuation is the realization of the self, the logical obsolescence of self-garbage necessarily comprises individuation as well. In a paradoxical way, the semanticized expression of this disconnection/disengagement is the sign of the one-way communication between the two levels of soul activity: the objective truth of their disengagement, implying the logical obsolescence of individuation and self as subjectivity, communicates itself to the disengaged subjective sphere through the semantics of self as discardable compacted brick of garbage.

Our dream is rooted in the present cultural and historical condition of the dreamer. This rootedness manifests itself in the first place in its semantic content, which is expressive of today's reality. As a rule, the images of the process of individuation in our time "do not represent the reality of the present",[97] due to the logical obsolescence of individuation, which "*is* the display of a former truth, but this display *itself* does not have the status of truth anymore".[98] Our dream seems to be one infinitesimal paradoxical exception to this rule: unless we abstract it from its real rootedness in the particular time and situation in which it occurs,

[96] Giegerich, *CEP V*, p. 334-335.
[97] Giegerich, *CEP V*, p. 342.
[98] Giegerich, *CEP V*, p. 343.

closing our eyes to the blatant correspondence between its central image and the objective truth of the logical obsolescence of self as subjectivity and of individuation, we must admit that the whole subjective situation represented in the dream is indicative of the *historical* locus of which it is expressive, and which *on principle* carries within itself the historical past, "both in sedimented form *as its own present real constitution* and as memory"—otherwise that locus could not be thought of as being *historical*.

We can give support to this conclusion from another angle: by definition, the self is not enclosed in the human individual, having an internal infinity of its own, an infinity that "does not have a *border* to the world, but rather *within itself* extends, and is open, to the community in which it lives, to the historical situation it finds itself in, and to the historical past it carries within itself (both in sedimented form as its own present real constitution and as memory)".[99] Consequently, the absolute negativity and internal infinity of self-as-garbage *on principle* communicates with the community and the historical situation it finds itself in. We could formulate the paradox of this dream by saying that precisely in depicting its own realm (that of *opus parvum*) as objectively obsolete, the dream is objectively up-to-date, it is a dream of the "*public, truly objective* 'objective psyche'".[100] It expresses semantically the obsolescence of the logic of the individual.

---

[99] Giegerich, *WIS*, p. 298-299. On a footnote to this passage, Giegerich states: "The I *is* its history."

[100] Giegerich, *CEP V*, p. 354. "Only if a young man's dream is not his individual dream, but if he is dreaming the Mercurial dream in today's

Returning to the dream-I's rejection of the initiation presented through the dream (similar to Jung's refusal to think the thought of the obsolescence of the notion of God),[101] we must admit that its reason (as in Jung's case) is in the adherence of the I to an already logically obsolete notion whose accomplished logical destruction is being depicted in the dream, as hinted at above. Looked at from a strictly *opus parvum* perspective, the dream-I could not endure the objective inner truth displayed in the dream because it meant the destruction of the grounds of her personal ego position at that moment. The dream-I resists this movement—or this thought—and this resistance is indicative of the moment of first or simple negation in the dialectical movement, in which there is "weeping and gnashing of teeth", as a result from a "dramatic clash": "the ego is turned from its partial views and illusions as it suffers what Jung calls the violence that is done to it by the Self".[102] But looked at from a deeper perspective, this logical violence is done to the entire subjective sphere, to soul as subject: the dream presents the devaluation of the entirety of the psy-

---

prime matter, in what is really going on in our time is it a dream of the objective psyche." (ibid., p. 352)

[101] To a modern humanist position of consciousness, it is as shocking to think of a shitting God as it is to think of self as garbage. What is at stake in both cases? A drastic negation of a previous notion of what "God" or "self" means, so that the devaluation manifested in the shocking semantic content is indicative of the ruin, if not necessarily of the notion itself, certainly of a particular expression of it, of a certain configuration of consciousness ruled by "God as sublime transcendent Being" and "self as the highest human value, *imago Dei*".

[102] Greg Mogenson, 'Different Moments in Dialectical Movement', in W. Giegerich, D. Miller and G. Mogenson. *Dialectics and Analytical Psychology. The El Capitan Canion Seminar*. New Orleans: Spring Journal and Books, 2005, p. 93.

chological difference in its all-too-human level, and precisely here it communicates with the soul truth of the age.

There is an important detail in the dream image which points to the logical condition of the specific historical locus in which it is produced. For the semantic expression of the *putrefactio* in the dream is not just in "garbage", but also in the particular form of "*compacted bricks*", which semantically moors the dream image in the specific form of life characteristic of *mass society*, giving to the alien-self the status not only of a common despicable matter, but of a *mass-produced* one. Mass production (in whatever form, even in the humble case of compacted bricks of garbage) is characteristic of our times. Therefore, the dream-I's rejection, directed to the whole process and not only to an aspect of it, reveals an opposition to the intrinsic *mass quality* of the produced self. Conversely, as the obsolescence of modern subjectivity—a stable logical feature of the objective soul in our time—is correlative of mass-mindedness, we can confirm from the mass quality attributed to the self-garbage that the syntactical moment of putrefaction in the dream's private process of individuation coincides with an essential aspect of the soul of the real. Hence, the dream-I is in opposition to the logic of mass mindedness. By extension, precisely due to this opposition, the dream-I must be thought of as being still partially influenced by a previous mindset, arguably of a humanist quality, in which consciousness *cannot* accept that "self"—its former highly valued essence—has logically decayed to nothing but "mass-produced garbage".

From this perspective, one can further understand the negative disgusted reaction of the dream-I: all the projects, values and views which she presumably stands by (in sum: her conscious position) are incompatible with an absolutely devalued discardable obsolete image of self. To follow the proposed path of initiation presented in the dream means "dying" to her present ego position. But dialectically envisaged, the truth of her present position is precisely that of "compacted bricks of garbage". In the dream she has ineluctably been expelled from the unconscious immersion in and protection from that truth. She is deprived of her previous idealized and obsolete views about (her)self and world. Self-garbage is the deeper truth of the superficial ego-level opinions and desires.

The dream thought exhibits an undeniable correspondence with the objective soul truth of the *logical obsolescence of soul as subjectivity or self*, a definitional feature of the logical form of Mass Man, as we saw. It is not difficult to establish a parallel between the devaluation implied in transforming people into compacted bricks of garbage and the truth of soul's *opus magnum* in the age of Technique and consumerism: the devaluation of personal human dimension is an objective aspect of the soul of the real. Human individuals are mere "inputs" to an impersonal objective process (which includes the superstructural ideology of presenting this process as existing in favor of those individuals, so that they willingly participate on it). They are *in truth* and from the outset expropriated from their former logically obsolete status (modern human subjects) and transformed into something new, other, precisely by being ascribed the logical status of Mass Man, *inasmuch as they are participants in the objective systems of the world.*[103] An empirical example may be helpful here.

Suppose the very ordinary situation of a teleseminar. While it happens, the participants are all connected to machines, to the technical apparatus. From the objective viewpoint (the viewpoint of the technical apparatus itself), their individualities are neither here nor there: they are not assimilated or needed by the objective apparatus, and as such they are *irrelevant* to the technical process going on at that moment. The participants' using (and giving themselves to) the objective technical process is all that counts objectively: they are merely *human impersonal input* to this process. The *truly* personal does not count in it. For instance: the effort in giving clear expression to a determinate thought in the teleseminar is objectively irrelevant if we consider the contents and meaning of the thought (which we may presume to be personal). It could be anything, it doesn't matter, as long as the effort in itself is sustained and feeds the technical process, making it alive (just as, in this very same moment, hundreds of millions of other human beings are making exactly the same thing, devoting themselves to the

[103] Jung compares the huge political and social organizations to a cancerous growth, because "they eat away man's nature as soon as they become ends in themselves and attain autonomy. From that moment they grow beyond man and escape his control. He becomes their victim and is sacrificed to the madness of an idea that knows no master. All the great organizations in which the individual no longer counts are exposed to this danger." (*CW* 10 § 719) Characteristically, he not only sees this situation as "madness", but also indicates his alternative to it: "There seems to be only one way of countering this threat to our lives, and that is the 'revaluation' of the individual." (ibid.) To Jung, the "global village" is nothing but a lunatic asylum, and its logic is helplessly and literally destructive of humankind, or "man's nature". The posthuman devaluation of the individual is categorically opposed in Jung's psychological project.

technical apparatus). On the other hand, from the subjective viewpoint, what is truly important is the expression of the contents and the production of meaning, or even better, the contents and meaning themselves. This dimension of the effort is part of one's larger personal movement of "becoming oneself".

Empirically speaking, by connecting oneself to the technical apparatus one establishes a *relation of continuity* between oneself and the apparatus. This *connection* creates a new situation in which the individual is integrated as a part of the technical environment *and* the technical environment is effectively realized, "brought into life", so to speak. In this new situation, *thought of from the point of view of the technical environment*, the personal individuality doesn't matter at all. It is irrelevant. All that counts is the information flowing "through the wires" from the individual to the "machines"; information that is grasped and algorithmically processed by the technical apparatus, which then executes its specific programmed task. In this way, the "machines" realize themselves, completely fulfilling their essence and purpose.

The personal subjective character of the individual is *useless* to the informational technical process. It has no function, no relevance. The individual connected as input to the technical apparatus can be anyone, regardless of race, gender, age, nationality, political profile, religious belief, socio-economic status, educational level, profession, personal history, aesthetic preferences, moral character etc. The human individuality is on principle discarded from the technical environment as irrelevant, and could be consistently imaged as "*garbage*": it has no use, no value for the process.[104] Hence we find an empirically available analogy for the logical identity of "*connecting*", "*compacting*" and "*transforming*" in the dream, of entering in relation to the technical apparatus and being transformed into "*compacted bricks of garbage*".

What distinguishes the modern form of consciousness from all other previous forms is its being *emancipated from soul*, its being equivalent to "born man". In the dream the self-garbage discardedness can be thought of as correlative of its emancipatedness. Therefore, the dream process may be interpreted as a first moment of an initiation into modern consciousness' *emancipatedness*. Correspondingly, from the standpoint of the soul of the real *today* an emancipated consciousness is superfluous, has no value or function at all, and thus is *logically* discardable, obsolete. And soul itself *produces* the conditions for emancipation, so that emancipation from soul does not mean stepping out of soul, but only a differentiation accomplished within soul itself.[105]

Now, in deepening this specific image of the self towards the logical place reserved to humanness in the ob-

[104] We could apply here what Wolfgang Giegerich says of information in a different context: "Information in the modern sense is *essentially* alienated from people, and people are alienated from it" (Giegerich, *CEP II*, p. 292)—even when this information is extracted from people.

[105] In a way, an emancipated self is not contained in soul anymore, it has been thrown out, so to speak. But it can only be emancipated if it has been devised by soul to be *discarded* from soul, which is also to say, if soul "wants" this emancipation (as a self-differentiation within itself), if *discardedness* is intrinsic to its logical constitution. Discardedness is here equivalent to logical obsolescence: the self is expressed in the dream as irrelevant garbage. But the question is: irrelevant to what? The ultimate answer is: to the objective sphere of soul's *opus magnum*.

jective order of the world today, we can see the paradox or ambiguity inherent to the logical status of Mass Man: it is the logical place where modern autonomous subjectivity finds its death (as we saw above, an empirical individual wholly engulfed by the logic of mass-mindedness is not an autonomous subject anymore). At the same time, this logical place is a gate to emancipation, *provided the individual consciousness acknowledges its objective sublatedness, obsolescence* (in the language of the dream: is initiated into its *objective* garbage status) so as to become able to differentiate itself from the logic of modern life, while at the same time participating on it as an atom in the mass. And it is precisely in fully and consciously surrendering itself to this logic that consciousness can be relatively freed of it, emancipating itself. The irrelevantification of all-too-human individual reality, its humiliating devaluation, forces consciousness to recognize the humble condition of the individual self-subject; in a similar way, Jung saw the "self" as the greatest limitation for man, "manifested in the experience: 'I am *only* that!'", the experience and consciousness of "our narrow confinement in the self".[106]

Due to the equivalence of the truth implied in the semantic depiction of self as "compacted brick of garbage" and the modern truth of the logical obsolescence of subjectivity, which precisely imposes the irrelevantification of human being, the logical obsolescence, sublatedness and sunkenness of subjectivity, it seems plausible to state that this small dream is *clearly* permeated and informed by the soul of the real. Consequently, the deeper psychological

[106] C.G.Jung. *MDR*, p. 325.

purpose of this dream is to initiate the dream-I into the modern truth into which the dreamer (and all of us) had been born and as which she consequently already existed.

To summarize my argument: my contention is that in the dream here presented there is arguably a disclosure of the hidden nature of the real, and thus in it there is a perceptible communication with the actual current status of soul at the level of *opus magnum*. As such, in this dream soul comes home to itself through the dream-I, initiating the individual consciousness into soul's objective *opus magnum* status. Hence my idea is that, in this case, the correspondence between the two separate levels is provided and realized by soul itself. While staying completely at the level of *opus parvum* (insofar as it is an *opus parvum* event, having only private *relevance*), the dream gives semantic expression to a truth belonging to the impersonal reality of soul's *opus magnum* (having thus objective *meaning*). This does not mean that it will have an inflated or spectacular relevance. No. It remains an all-too-human objectively irrelevant event, as such only relevant to the individual subject living it. It only follows the logical patterns of the historical locus in which it occurs; this is what constitutes its broader interest to us. And this embeddedness in the soul of the real can even have a disinflating effect, insofar as it cannot be seen as being original, one-of-a-kind, but is only that: a normal psychic event liable to happen to many people in this time and age. No big deal.

Maybe, when and if consciousness is able to assume the logical obsolescence of its former highest value—Man—and realistically acknowledge the new post-human dominant higher soul value—Technology—, it will not be so shocking for the empirical individual to see subjectivity represented as garbage *in relation to the broader inhuman organization of the world*: it may be the humiliating way of reaching now the position of recognizing one's true size: "I'm only that". Paradoxically, it may also be the way of breaking the identification with the logic of our new modern life and of returning to the humble human condition, to the logical obsolescence of the subjective truth. Through this differentiation one is freed to cultivate one's own subjectivity according to the logically obsolete ideals of humanism, engaging oneself in the logically humble ways of individuation—objectively obsolete, but perhaps existentially, subjectively indispensable to many people. Soul's *opus magnum* will not be affected by this private, subjective possibility. Culture will not be "healed". The world will follow its historical destiny. No inflated salvationist heroism here. The fully accomplished emancipation from soul, which has to be consciously performed through the initiation of the individual in the soul truth of our age, is thus the only possible way of avoiding the sheer and total coincidence of personal subjective reality and objective logical status of Mass Man. Objectively, the logical form of trash-subjectivity is inescapable; subjectively, it does not have to be literalized.[107]

[107] "All the new technical and scientific developments do not have to go to our heads. I do not need to personally embrace every new technical possibility and to get enthralled and engulfed by a fascination for it as if it entailed the promise of heaven on earth, nor do I have to personally identify with the logic of modernity and thus forget who I really am and what my real needs as a human being are. But on the other hand, I certainly do want to stay aware of and in contact with the soul's *opus magnum* and respect and appreciate it. I see the obsolescence, sublatedness,

sunkenness of what may be of great importance to me as private individual. (…) But then again, I also keep my distance from it, distinguish and emancipate myself from where the soul is today, from the new logic of modern life, holding my place and staying down to earth as '*only* that!,' living my life *only* as this private individual that I am, in conscious recognition of my human-all-too-humanness and my personal needs as a human being." (Giegerich, *CEP V,* p. 368)

ABOUT THE AUTHOR

Marco Heleno Barreto (Brazil), PhD, is a Jungian psychotherapist, working in private practice. He teaches philosophy at FAJE – Faculdade Jesuíta de Filosofia e Teologia, in Belo Horizonte, Brazil. He is the author of *Símbolo e Sabedoria Prática. C.G. Jung e o Mal-estar da Modernidade* (2008), *Imaginação Simbólica. Reflexões Introdutórias* (2008), *Pensar Jung* (2012), *Homo imaginans. A imaginação criadora na estética de Gaston Bachelard* (2016) and *Estudos (Pós)Junguianos* (2018). He also has contributed articles to *Spring Journal*, *International Journal of Jungian Studies*, *Journal of Analytical Psychology* and *Jung Journal*. He presently serves on the Executive Committee of the International Society for Psychology as the Discipline of Interiority (ISPDI).

Made in United States
Troutdale, OR
11/03/2026

56845258R00066